FROM
VICTIM
TO VICTOR

FROM
VICTIM
TO VICTOR

BOB WELLS

XULON PRESS

Xulon Press
2301 Lucien Way #415
Maitland, FL 32751
407.339.4217
www.xulonpress.com

Printed in the United States of America.

Paperback ISBN-13: 978-1-66280-561-5
eBook ISBN-13: 978-1-6628-0562-2

Dedication

I DEDICATE THIS BOOK TO GOD THE FATHER, THE Son, and the Holy Spirit. I can do all things through Christ which strengthens me, and I can do nothing apart from Him. Writing this book is proof of this truth. I also dedicate this book to my spicy rib, my Babe, my wife, Cathy Wells. We are one and we have done and will do life together. I love you so much, you are Cathy to the infinity to me! Finally, I dedicate this book to all the people that want to break free from habits, addictions, and strongholds. My prayer is that you will daily recognize when the victim mentality is holding you back and you will apply the concepts in this book to live as a Victor!

Acknowledgments

First of all, I want to acknowledge my Lord and Savior Jesus Christ. You helped me believe I am a Victor! You pushed me to stop making excuses (accepting a victim mentality). You carry me when I get discouraged and want to quit. Most of all, I thank You that You are my friend and You stick closer than a brother. Thank You, Jesus.

I also want to acknowledge my beautiful wife, Cathy, for encouraging me to write this book. I thank you for giving me a reason to want to be healthy. I am so in love with you and I look forward to decades of healthy life and love together.

To my children, The Welzies, WOW! I'm a **blessed** man! Every day I thank God for each of you. Robert, Bobcat, Detroit!; you XL. You choose the harder right and nothing deters you because you are a Victor. Thank you and Lynn for Stormy Claire, a most beautiful reason for me to get healthy. Alexis, Lexi, she's my Lexi Wells, pretty girl, she's so beautiful, and I love her so, don't you know? I love ya to the juv ya, bada, bada bing bang, boomp! You are full of compassion and the world is a better place because of you are a Victor! Caleb, Bubba Bear, you are tenacious, you never quit. Handsome, intelligent, athletic, a great dancer, and you are funny. All that adds up to you are a

Victor! Moriah Renee, Monee, Bootsy Scooter a lot of girls look good, but Bootsy is cuter, you'd say the same thing if you knew her. You set your goal and you far exceed it, ORU, Barnabas, RN, BSN. The world is yours because you are a Victor! Analee Simone, Analita, Analee, Analee how oh how are you, Analee, Analee you oh you're so cute. Analee, Analee I like you, yes I do, I like you! The Great Comeback, Captain of the team, incredible saves, smart, beautiful, great dancer, fashionista, you got a life, a victorious life!

To my Dad and Mom, Bob and Alice Wells. The greatest parents ever! Mom, I will always love my Mama! I miss you and I know I will see you in Heaven, your stories, your love of people, and your faith in God continue to inspire me. Dad, you are my **hero**! I know how to love because I've seen you demonstrate it! Thank you for being a great role model for men in general, and me and my sons in particular. To my sisters, especially my favorite, and you know who you are. Yes, Alison, Kim, and Rae you are my favorite. Thank you each for encouraging me to finish this book. I love y'all.

This is hard because so many people have helped me and encouraged me. My Summit Church family—Pastors Rick and Cindy Godwin, Percy and Daynelle Kikmbrough, Gary Pinion, My Wednesday Night Men's Group—DG, EBM, CW, Doc, TR, MB, and all the "fellas." I love you brothers and I finally got "a round to it!" Legacy of Love Marriage Ministry Team—I want to acknowledge these pastors and leaders that have helped me directly and indirectly: Pastor Archie Neal,

Pastor Thomas Miller, Pastor Larry Stockstill, Minister George Rose, Kenneth and Gloria Copeland, George Pearsons, Creflo Dollar, Bill Winston, Jesse Duplantis, Jerry Savelle, Bishop TD Jakes, Joseph Prince, and so many others that I listened to as I walked daily and lost over 100 pounds. Matt Lara—"What you got? Get you some! What's the Holy Spirit speaking to you today?" I love you my brother!

Finally, thank you to the Xulon Press Team, especially Gina Fleming and Dr. Larry Keefauver. Dr. Larry, after each edit, I would tell my wife I wanted to buy this book. I am so grateful to you Dr. Larry and your encouragement has stirred me to continue to live as a Victor.

TABLE OF CONTENTS

PREFACE

Choose Life

> *"I call heaven and earth to witness against you today, that I have set before you life and death, blessing and curse. Therefore **choose life**, that you and your offspring may live, loving the Lord your God, obeying his voice and holding fast to him, for he is your life and length of days, that you may dwell in the land that the Lord swore to your fathers, to Abraham, to Isaac, and to Jacob, to give them."* (Deuteronomy 30:19-20 ESV)

I'm writing this book to help others realize that being a **victim** is a choice and so is being a **Victor**! I have had a wonderful life compared to many other people. My parents are awesome! They raised me and my wonderful sisters with love, care, and attention. My Dad is my hero. He worked hard, he talked with me, and played ball with me. He led our family, he took us to church, provided a home, food, and clothing. He will quickly correct me that God provided those things and he is so thankful for all God has done and is doing.

I'll always love my Mama, she brought me in this world. My Mom was always an encourager! She was the neighborhood's favorite mom. Everybody was blessed when they were around her. My Mom passed away before I finished writing this book. I love her and my memory of her inspires me to finish this book and reach my goal of weighing 180 pounds.

My parents were role models for me of how to love, how to be married, and how to enjoy that marriage! What has that got to do with moving from being a victim to a victor? Everything, because I chose to be a victim! I could just as easily have chosen to be a victor. Other people have come from backgrounds much worse than mine and made a choice **not** to allow circumstances to dictate how they would live. Others have made a choice to blame people, events, tragedies, and circumstances for their lot in life. I have not been through those circumstances; I have not dealt with those issues. I know they haunt you and taunt you!

I am not going to tell you that choosing to be a **Victor** is easy. I am telling you that **you** "must" choose to be a **Victor** if you want to succeed in this life! One of my favorite Scriptures is in Deuteronomy 30:19-20, spoken to God's people who had been slaves for 400 years. "I call heaven and earth to witness against you today, that I have set before you life and death, blessing, and curse. Therefore **choose life**, that you and your offspring may live, loving the Lord your God, obeying his voice and holding fast to him, for he is your life and length of days, that you may dwell in the land that the Lord swore to your fathers, to Abraham, to Isaac, and to Jacob, to give them" (ESV emphasis added).

My wife loves to note that God recognizes that this could be a tough pop quiz for some of us, so He gives us the answer, "Choose Life!" My point is, God promises that you "can" choose life. At any moment, you can make the choice! No devil or evil spirit can stop you, **none**! The biggest, best decision/choice you can make is the choice to make Jesus Christ your Lord and Savior. If the devil could stop you from making any decision, this would be the one, but he doesn't because he can't! You choose, God cannot stop you from making the wrong choice, so the devil can't stop you from making the right choice!

Choose life and choose to be a Victor.

I started writing this a couple of months after I made the choice to be a **Victor** in my weight and health. My journey began at 363 pounds and will continue as I get my weight down to 180 pounds and maintain a healthy weight for the rest of my life; my long satisfying life! I am going to share the wisdom God gave me as I started, continued, pressed through, and obtained my goal. My focus in this book is on choosing to be a victor instead of a victim. I will use my weight loss and health improvement as an example of how I did that. I know that the principles can be applied to several areas of life, like finances, marriage, parenting, etc.

"The remarkable thing is, we have a choice every day regarding the attitude we will embrace for that day."- Chuck Swindoll[1]

Oh, God, I need a do-over! I need to do my whole life over! Look at this mess! Oh, God! I have made a mess out of my life! Father, I am a failure! Look at me, a West Point graduate, Army infantry officer, and I'm over 360 pounds! I'm in debt, I'm not able to pay my bills, I'm a tither and a giver, and I'm struggling from paycheck to paycheck! My wife has to work. I have failed as a father! My oldest children have turned from pursuing You! I'm called into the ministry and I'm afraid to do what you have called me to do! I go through the motions as a marriage counselor, as a men's ministry leader, as a teacher! God! Help me! Help me! God, I have ruined my life and wasted the gifts and talents you blessed me with. I want a do-over!

Chapter 1

Victim vs. Victor

God, I have ruined my life and wasted the gifts and talents You blessed me with. I want a do-over! This was my prayer several days per week on my drive home from work for about 18 months. I knew I was better than the fruit my life was producing, and I knew **I** was the problem! I did not know that this prayer was the start of God's restoration in my life. For years, I had "complain" prayed.

> *"God, why can't I eat a bunch of junk food, sit on my butt,*
> *and lose weight?" "God, why do You bless people that*
> *don't tithe, who don't even think about You,*
> *but they have millions?"*
> *"God, we have kept our kids from celebrating all the devil-in-*
> *spired movies,*
> *music, Halloween, and the Easter bunny!*
> *Why are they running from following You?"*
> *"God, why am I such a victim?"*

Ask Yourself…

Have I ever "complain" prayed?
How did that work out for me?

That is the key!
For years, I saw myself as a victim
of situations and circumstances.

I saw myself "trying" to get God to bless me and to help me. In my eyes, events were holding me back, keeping me down, overpowering, and overwhelming me. I was a victim of circumstance. (Some of you Three Stooges fans might recognize that phrase). I was living my life as a victim. I was accepting my position and my lot in life as God's will for me. It was no use trying to improve. I kind of tried and it didn't work, so why keep trying?

I tried to change my diet for a couple of weeks, but my wife, Cathy, would cook something not on my diet and I "had" to eat it! I tried working out for a couple of weeks, but I had to get to work on time and by the time I got up and drove to the gym/fitness center at work, I only had 20 minutes. So, I had to go get a couple of breakfast tacos instead!

"Oh God, why am I getting so big? My 3XL shirts are tight and my size 52 waist pants are tight, why God?" Go ahead laugh. Looking at it now, I see how foolish I was, but I was sincerely convinced that God was conspiring against me to keep me messed up. I reasoned that I must have done something to displease God, so my weight, my finances, my marriage, my kids, and my life were supposed to be a mess. I was a victim. A 360-pound victim!

I realized that I was choosing to be a victim when I was praying for God to help me because I listened to Frank Sinatra and I had done it my way. What a hot mess! I was particularly ashamed of my weight and health. I was 363 pounds by the time I got up the courage to weigh myself. I probably weighed more than that, but weighing over 300 pounds is a mess, so 363 pounds is a huge mess.

If you looked at me and my life from the outside, you would have thought it was good. I was a master of deception. I put on the "I'm blessed and highly favored!" make-up face like a trained Hollywood professional! Inside, I was hurting, I was dying, and I was crying when nobody was looking! I knew I had to do something.

Romans 7 and 8

I chose to turn to the Word of God! The answer to every need is in the Bible. Romans 8:1 is my absolute favorite scripture in the Bible. I leaned on Romans chapter 7 for years as an excuse for giving in to pornography. I would read Paul's words and I could identify with his struggle. I didn't want to look at that filth, I hated it and myself, but I did it anyway! I would excuse myself, though, by reasoning that I was just struggling like the great Apostle Paul had struggled.

Then I would read Romans 8:1, "There is, therefore, now, no condemnation for those who are in Christ Jesus." Glory to God, Hallelujah to Jesus! I'm not going to hell. God is not condemning me! However, I didn't get an understanding of the next two verses for a very long time. In Romans 8:2-3, Paul tells us that we are free from the authority, power, and ownership of sin! Before I became a Christian, I **had** to obey sin. Sin owned me, sin was my king, my ruler. But once I chose to make Jesus the Lord, the King, the Ruler of my life, I was set free from **all** the power and control of sin! Glory to God! I can choose not to sin. I can tell sin no! I can choose to obey God! This revelation hit a nerve. I could choose not to be obese! However, that's not the whole equation for success.

Pastor Rick Godwin, teaches, exhorts, and challenges us to stop curling up in the fetal position, sucking our thumbs, and waiting for God or somebody else to do it for us.

We must get up, trust God, and make the changes we need to make to bring God glory by our success. I wanted to obey, and like lots of other things I wanted to do, I was just wishfully thinking. Then I started listening with an ear to hear to the teachings by Kenneth Copeland. In one particular message, Brother Copeland talked about how he read Philippians 2:13, "for it is God who works in you both to will and to do for His good pleasure" (NKJV). Brother Copeland explained that God will help us want or will or desire to do His will! On top of that,

God will give us the power, the ability, the skills, and the knowledge to then DO His will! So, since we now want to do His will and He has empowered us TO DO His will, Philippians 4:13 says, "I can do all things through Christ who strengthens me" (NKJV). Brother Copeland said he started praying, "Lord, I'm willing to be willing!" I thought it made logical sense, so I started praying, "Lord, I'm willing to be willing!"

Ask Yourself...
Am I willing to be willing to do His will?

It was during this time of developing a closer walk with my Lord that He gave me a revelation of choosing to be a victim or a victor. The Lord began to give me an outline for this book. I wrote down the outline and then I realized that in order to credibly endorse the principles, I needed a victory. Hmmm, what to do? So, this writing sat for almost 2 years while I tried to figure it out. I didn't have a Damascus road experience, but one day I felt the Lord prompt me that making a 180-degree life turn is what I needed to lose weight. Then I thought, "Hey, I'm probably about 360 pounds. I can go from 360 pounds to 180 pounds and that would be a victory!" That revelation came about 8 months before I started to write this book and a couple of months before I embarked on my weight loss journey. I lost 60 pounds in 5 months by November of 2015. Since this is a work in progress, by December of 2016, I had lost 120 pounds. In March of 2018, I gained 40 pounds, but I am a victor and not a victim, so by the time I get this book published, I will have lost 180 pounds!

Defining Victor and Victim

I consider Pastor Archie Neal my spiritual father. He likes to provide definitions in his teaching messages. It helps us better understand what is being taught. So, I want to start by defining our two positions, **Victor** and **Victim**. One definition of "victor" is a person who defeats an enemy or opponent in a battle, game, or other competition. The definition of "victim" is a person harmed, injured, or killed, as a result of a crime, accident, or other event or action. A person who is tricked or duped. A person who is deceived or cheated, as by his own emotions or ignorance, by the dishonesty of others, or by some impersonal agency. One definition of "victim mentality" is an acquired (learned) personality trait in which a person tends to regard himself as a victim of the negative actions of others, and to think, speak, and act as if that were the case--even in the absence of clear evidence.[2]

The Lord brought it to my attention that victor and victim are only different by the last two letters. So, I looked up the root "vict." I found it is derived from the Latin "vincere," which means "to conquer." It can also be linked to the Old English "Weik," which means " to fight, conquer." I also found an Old Norwegian root "vigr," which means "able in battle." So, using the root definitions, to conquer, to fight, able in battle," and adding the suffix "or" I derived that a vict(or) is one who conquers in a fight, one who is able in battle. In contrast, adding the suffix "im" means a vict(im) is one who is conquered in a fight, one incapable in battle.

My struggle was I enjoyed being a victim. I nurtured my victim mentality. Being a victim allowed me to avoid taking responsibility for my life. Being a victor required me to take responsibility for my life. Being a victim allowed me to forget the poor choices I made/make. Being a victor required me to recognize I have made choices that affect my life. I chose to do or not to do, I chose to say or not to say, I chose! I believe being a victor or a victim is a choice.

Good things happen and bad things happen, a victor thrives in either situation while a victim suffers in either situation. I'm not talking about being self-reliant, but realizing, believing, and trusting God that no matter what, I can do **all** things through Him, no matter what. He causes **all** things to work together for good, no matter what. I have overcome them by the blood of the Lamb. I have found so many Scriptures that explain where the strength to choose to be a victor comes from and I will share them as we proceed through this book.

The Blame Game

I lived for over thirty years blaming other people, circumstances, situations (both under my control and outside of my control), and even God for my failures in life! Yes, I blamed

God! "Why did He let me...? Why didn't He do a miracle? Why didn't He bless my decisions?" I know I'm the only person who has thought that way. I blamed my precious wife! She doesn't want me to stay after work to exercise, she won't cook healthy food, she doesn't believe I'm called to the ministry, she won't exercise with me. I blamed my kids, they need the new game, and they need me to go to this event. I blamed my mom and dad. I blamed West Point because I went Infantry instead of Field Artillery, I could have been fat in Field Artillery and stayed in the Army. I blamed the bosses when I did not get promoted! Well, I will show them, "I will do an average job in this position that is far below my skills and qualifications!" I blamed anybody but Robert Lee Wells Jr!

Ask Yourself...

What and who have I blamed for my failures in life?

I know it's foolish and I hope after you stop laughing you will consider if you have made any similar excuses. I know there are a couple of other expert excuse-makers, professionals at the Blame-game out there! I learned, though, that no one wins the Blame-game. The Blame-game has no winners! You cannot succeed in the Excuse-making industry. What is produced is always a loss, a defeat! The most beautiful excuse ever produced is worthless. The excuse is offered to explain why you failed. The excuse doesn't turn the failure into a victory. Stop playing the Blame-game. Leave the Excuse-making industry. Decide to take responsibility for your choices. Recognize and own up to your part in the situation, problem, or failure.

I finally realized that to be a victor, I had to own my problems and my failures. Be careful here, though, I don't consider myself a failure or a problem. I may have a problem and I may experience a failure, but I am not either of those. I am a child of God. I am the righteousness of God in Christ Jesus. I ate too much fattening, unhealthy food, but I'm not going to label myself as an unhealthy over-eater. Because as the Bible says, "For as he thinks in his heart, so is he..." (Proverbs 23:7 NKJV). I would sit and watch TV instead of exercising, I would sleep when I should get up to read the Bible, pray, and go exercise. I thought I was lazy and unproductive. When I believed and agreed with that, I easily became a 360-pound obese man.

I had to change my thinking to change my life, but how? The Lord showed me. By using the first four letters (V-I-C-T) of "victor" and "victim" and contrasting the last two letters (OR and IM), I changed my thinking and changed my life! The Lord gave me three traits/characteristics of each of the first four letters. As I applied and continue to apply these lessons, I am becoming a victor and overcoming the victim mentality.

I thought I had finished this book at the end of September 2017. I asked my pastor, Rick Godwin to give it a cursory read. He did and said he thought it was good and with a few changes could be published. I was excited and immediately sat down to do it. However, I soon stopped working on this book and stopped looking at my goal of being 180 pounds. I gained twenty pounds. I could try to blame the winter holidays or busyness of work or any of the other excuses we like to use. However, I made a conscious choice and resumed working on the book and my quest to achieve my goal. I may not be 180 pounds at that publishing of this book, but I will get healthier every day and I will reach my goal because I am a victor, not a victim.

Chapter Review

At the end of each chapter, I suggest you take a few minutes and review the **Ask Yourself** questions and the **Key Points** highlighted in this chapter. Also, take the time to read and meditate on the **scriptures** that helped me on my journey from **Victim** to **Victor**.

Ask Yourself...
Have I ever "complain" prayed?
How did that work out for me?

Ask Yourself...
*Am I willing to be willing to **do** His will?*

Ask Yourself...
What and who have I blamed for my failures in life?

Key Points Review:

➢ Choose life and choose to be a **Victor.**

➢ For years, I saw myself as a victim of situations and circumstances.

➢ Pastor Rick Godwin teaches, exhorts, and challenges us to stop curling up in the fetal position, sucking our thumbs, and waiting for God or somebody else to do it for us.

Record what God reveals to you from each of these scriptures:

Deuteronomy 30:19-20
Romans 8:1-3
Philippians 2:13
Philippians 4:13
Proverbs 23:7

Pray and ask God to open your heart and mind to receive His truth as you proceed through this study of moving from **Victim** to **Victor.**

Part i

V

The " **V** " in **Victor** looks at, understands, and listens to three traits: Vision, Value, and Voice. I had to make adjustments in all three of these traits in order to move forward from a victim to a **Victor** mindset. I had to seek God's Vision for my life in general and my health in particular. I had to understand my Value to God, to my family, and to the world. I had to value my life, my family, my health, and my purpose. I had to screen the Voices I listened to. I had to change what I voiced about myself, my health, and my life.

I have to continue to see the Vision, hear and speak the Voice of Victory, understand my Value, and place Value on my life. The "V's" are where we start to think, talk, act, and live like a **Victor**. The life of Caleb provides an excellent model of how the "V's" can help us become a **Victor**. Let's begin by looking at Vision in the life of Caleb.

Chapter 2

Vision

A dictionary definition of Vision is: the ability to see; sight or eyesight; something that you imagine; a picture that you see in your mind; something that you see or dream especially as part of a religious or supernatural experience.[3] The basic premise of Vision is that, "what you see is what you get." If you keep looking at and focusing on your problems, your deficiencies, your lack, your sickness, and your failures, then you will keep having those problems, those deficiencies, that lack, that sickness, and that failure. Often, they even grow and multiply!

Ask Yourself...

Have I been focusing on my problems, deficiencies, my lack, and my failures?

How has that been working out for me?

The truth is God did not create anyone to be a failure! God created each of us to be blessed so we can in turn be a blessing. When you get saved, born again, and accept Jesus as your Lord and Savior, God creates a **new you**! Old things pass away, and

all things become new (2 Corinthians 5:17). The "failure" died and the blessing is made alive. If you are born again, you **are** a blessing. See yourself that way. See yourself as an overcomer. See yourself as more than a conqueror. See yourself as a **Victor!**

Ask Yourself…

Do I see myself as an overcomer, more t han a conqueror, and a blessing to others?

If the answer is no, why not?

Why Is Vision Important to a Victor?

> *"Now then, just as the LORD promised, he has kept me alive for forty-five years since the time he said this to Moses, while Israel moved about in the wilderness. So here I am today, eighty-five years old! I am still as strong today as the day Moses sent me out; I'm just as vigorous to go out to battle now as I was then. Now give me this hill country that the LORD promised me that day. You yourself heard then that the Anakites were there and their cities were large and fortified, but, the LORD helping me, I will drive them out just as he said."* (Joshua 14:10-12 NIV).

Looking at the impact of **Vision** in Caleb's life, we see that having a **Vision** did four things:

1. It gave him **focus**.
2. It gave him an **aim**.
3. It filled him with **passion**.
4. It kept him **alive**.

Victors, like Caleb, don't look for an easy way, a quick way, or the path of least resistance.

Victors win! That is why we are called Victors.

It doesn't matter what we face, we **win**! We are **Victors**! Do I make it sound like we should never believe any problem is too difficult? Yes, because Jesus already faced and endured every problem, issue, and fear that we could ever encounter, and **He won**! He then placed the championship belt, the trophy, and the gold medal on each of His believers. God says we share Jesus' victory just as if we had won it.

You must see that. You need to have a **Vision** of your complete victory. You have to see yourself as a **Victor**, because as that prophet of old, Flip Wilson used to say, "What you see is what you get!"

Focus: So, one of the most compelling reasons to get God's vision of you and your life is to **focus** on where you are going. Caleb was focused on getting his mountain. He could see that mountain and thought about the home he would build on that mountain. He could see his grandchildren and great-grandchildren living on that mountain. Many of the people around him grumbled and complained, but not Caleb. He kept saying he was getting that mountain. He kept that mountain in focus.

When there was not enough water, he thought about the water running down that mountain. When they needed food, he thought about the deer on that mountain. When enemies attacked the children of Israel, he thought about how he was going to cut down giants on his mountain. He was focused!

I must focus. When I only lose a pound after a week of intense exercise, I need to think about how I am going to be able to do even more intense exercise when I am 180 pounds. When I eat a slice of pizza instead of a grilled chicken breast, I think about how I will desire healthful foods when I am 180 pounds. I have to keep the vision of my 180-pound life in the front of my mind.

Ask Yourself...

What do I need to do to keep my focus on my God-given vision in the front of my mind?

Aim: The Vision gave Caleb something to **aim** for. Wandering through the desert and going around a mountain that is not your mountain can cause anyone to forget why they started on the journey in the first place. Caleb told Joshua, "You remember the word Moses, the Man of God, spoke to me..." Caleb was aiming for that mountain. One week after Moses told him that he would get the mountain, Caleb was pumped and a month later, he was still pumped. A year later, he was still pumped. A decade later, Caleb was still aiming to get that mountain. Thirty years later, Caleb said, "I'm still kicking butt and taking names! I'm getting that mountain!" Forty years later, Caleb said, "Let me practice on these baby giants, so, I can be ready for the giants trespassing on my mountain!"[4]

I know I am going to get to 180 pounds. Setbacks may happen, delays may occur, but like Caleb and the Apostle Paul, I say, "Brethren, I do not count myself to have apprehended; but one thing I do, forgetting those things which are behind and reaching forward to those things which are ahead, I press toward the goal for the prize of the upward call of God in Christ Jesus" (Philippians 3:13-14 NKJV).

My aim drives me to keep going until I reach my goal.

Passion: The focus and aim stirred up a passion in Caleb. How do I know he had passion? Because forty-five years later, he is still holding onto that Word. Forty-five years later, he says he is as strong at eighty-five as he was at forty. When other people were grumbling and complaining, he was steadfast in his passion to get his mountain.

As I think about and work toward getting down to 180 pounds, I know that a passion is stirred up inside of me. I need to get down to 180 pounds. I see myself with a muscular body, with clothes that fit, playing with my grandkids, and running 10Ks and triathlons. I have a passion. It's taken longer than I wanted it to, and that is mostly my fault, but the vision of being healthy and weighing 180 pounds has given me the passion to accomplish something many people considered impossible for Bob Wells to do. I have to stir up that passion daily and I will get to my goal.

Ask Yourself...

What do I need to do to continually stir up the passion to move forward toward my God-given vision?

Alive: Finally, the **Vision** kept Caleb alive. He was not just breathing, not just existing, but **alive** and refusing to go quietly into the night. Caleb woke up every morning believing this is **the** day, and if it is not **the** day, it is getting me one day closer to **the** day. Regardless, I am **alive** and I will get my mountain! I can see Caleb talking to his sons and daughter about the mountain, about living on the mountain, about the fruit and lushness of the mountain. I can see him talking to his grandchildren and having them tell him about taking down the giants on **their** mountain. I hear that in his words, "Now then, just as the Lord promised, he has kept me alive for forty-five years since the time he said this to Moses..."]

You are probably asking, "How do I get a **Vision** of myself as a **Victor**? I look in the mirror and I see me. I know that person is not a victor. I know all too well the problems, failures, and issues of that person in the mirror. How do I get a **Vision** of myself as more than a conqueror, as a **Victor**?" I'm glad you asked.

First, pray and ask God to show you a vision of the real you. Ask Him for a vision of the new creation you. Ask Him for a vision of how He sees you.

Jesus says: "Ask, and it will be given to you; seek, and you will find; knock, and it will be opened to you. For everyone who asks receives, and he who seeks finds, and to him who knocks it will be opened...If you then, being evil, know how to give good gifts to your children, how much more will your Father who is in heaven give good things to those who ask Him!" (Matthew 7:7-8, 11 NKJV).

Ask Yourself...

Have I prayed and asked God for the vision of how He sees me? What did He show me?

God showed me a picture of myself 120 pounds lighter and He told me I would ask my wife, "What are you gonna do with me like this girl?" By November of 2016, I had lost 120 pounds, I did ask her, and she answered. So, I only had 60 pounds to go, glory to God!

This book is not a study on how to get an answer to prayer. However, I did learn to apply Mark 11:22-24:

1. Have **faith** in God.
2. **Pray** for all things.
3. **Speak** to whatever mountain I'm facing.
4. **Believe** I receive what I'm praying for.

5. **Forgive** others and myself.

Believe you receive the Vision and forgive yourself and anyone that has blurred, obscured, or deterred your Vision.

Chapter Review

I suggest you take a few minutes and review the **Ask Yourself** questions and the **Key Points** highlighted in this chapter. Also, take the time to read and meditate on the **scriptures** that helped me on my journey from **Victim** to **Victor**.

Ask Yourself…

Have I been focusing on my problems, deficiencies, my lack, and my failures?

How has that been working out for me?

Ask Yourself…

Do I see myself as an overcomer, more than a conqueror, and a blessing to others?

If the answer is no, why not?

Ask Yourself…

What do I need to do to keep my focus on my God-given vision in the front of my mind?

Ask Yourself...

What do I need to do to continually stir up the passion to move forward toward my God-given vision?

Ask Yourself...

Have I prayed and asked God for the vision of how He sees me? What did He show me?

Key Points Review:

➢ **Victors win! That is why we are called Victors.**

➢ **My aim drives me to keep going until I reach my goal.**

➢ **Believe you receive the Vision and forgive yourself and anyone that has blurred, obscured, or deterred your Vision.**

Record what God reveals to you from each of these scriptures:

2 Corinthians 5:17

Joshua 14:10-12

Philippians 3:13-14

Matthew 7:7-8, 11

Mark 11:22-24

Pray and ask God for a vision of you healed, healthy, wealthy, in a great marriage, raising godly children, etc. Have faith in

God that He has a vision for you and that He will show it to you. Pray for the eyes of your spirit to be opened so you can see!

CHAPTER 3

VALUE

CALEB VALUED THE PROMISE OF GOD THROUGH
Moses and he did not let go of that promise! I know that I
have given up on goals like losing weight because I tried really
hard for a couple of days and I gained weight. I did not value
reaching the goal or achieving success enough to push through.
Caleb had to go through day after day of hearing murmuring,
complaining, doubt, and rebellion. He watched as family and
friends passed away. He fought in battles with Joshua and forty-five years later, just as if it were the next day, Caleb reminds
Joshua of the promise. He valued that promise.

Caleb valued his life, his purpose, and God.

Therefore, my next step in moving from victim to **Victor**
was to begin to Value my life, my God-given purpose, and God.
I thought I valued myself because I fed myself and rested myself
and tried to avoid stressing myself. I thought I valued my purpose because I helped at church, got involved in marriage ministry, and went to the men's meetings. I thought I valued people

because I only cursed idiots that didn't know how to drive, referees that made stupid calls, or people that called in for ridiculously stupid reasons. I tried to keep my yard mowed. I thought I valued God because I prayed from time to time, tithed, and read the Bible frequently. I asked God for things and to bless my plan. I obeyed God when I could. OUCH!

Ask Yourself...

How do I show that I value my life, my God-given purpose, and God?

Do I truly value these important areas of my life?

Yes, I thought I valued these important areas of my life, but let's look at a definition of value. As a noun, it means the regard that something is held to deserve; the importance, worth, or usefulness of something; a person's principles or standards of behavior; one's judgment of what is important in life. As a verb, it is defined as estimated monetary worth of (something); consider (someone or something) to be important or beneficial; have a high opinion of.[5]

The word **Value**, like many words in the English language, can be a noun or a verb. When I think about value, I think about the noun tense of my verb application. In other words, are my actions confirming my intentions? I want to value God, my life, my purpose, my family, and other people. The intent and desire are there, but I must put action behind my intentions. My actions demonstrate the level of value I have for God, my life, my purpose, my family, etc. I realized that the only level that matters and gets results is high value. A low level of value is really "no" value.

Ask Yourself...
What are my high-level values?
What are my low-level values?

When too many other things come along that we place a higher value on, lowly valued items get pushed aside. For instance, if I place a low level of value on lawn care, if a comedy that I have seen before comes on TV, since I have assigned a high level of value on pleasure and comfort, I let the weeds and grass grow. Yes, I know that a week later, because I value the opinion of my neighbors and the HOA, I will have to do more work, but at that moment in time, my values are not prioritized.

If I assign a low-level of value to my marriage, then I will do a minimum to stay out of divorce court, but I won't work to make my marriage flourish! I may think I place a high level of value on my marriage because I agree to take my wife to a movie next Friday. However, if my buddy calls me and says he has an extra ticket to a Spurs playoff game with access to his company suite, and I call my wife to present her with my dilemma, she doesn't see the problem. I'm thinking Spurs versus chick-flick. She thinks her versus my buddy. Who do I want to be with more?

Getting back to weight loss, if I say I place a high level of value on being healthy, but I sit around eating chips and cookies and drinking sodas and milkshakes, well, I don't really value being healthy. I'm fooling myself if I say I value being healthy, but I continue doing things that ruin my health. I remember thinking that if I had a fit, well-defined muscular body, then I would eat better and exercise more. I'm serious! I thought if I had a body like my sons, I would want to eat salad and grilled chicken and I wouldn't eat cakes, chips, and candy bars. I would go to the gym and workout and run. If I were fit, I would value being fit! Thankfully, the Lord said, "Bob, you do realize that the reason your sons are fit and have chiseled bodies is because they value fitness?" Light bulbs popped. If I value fitness and good health, I will eat right and exercise and eventually I will get a fit body.

The Value Statement

The Lord helped me with assigning true value with what I call the Value Statement. The Value Statement has this format: I am _____, I deserve _____, and I am obligated to _____. It is important to put the right thing in the "I am" section. I am healthy, I am an excellent husband/spouse, I am a Christian, I am an excellent employee, etc.

The point is that I say I am what I desire to be and not what I think I am right now. On my weight loss journey from victim to victor, the first part of the Value Statement is I am a 180-pound fit man. I know that ten out of ten scales will report that

I am not a 180-pound man, fit or otherwise. I am not basing my "I am" statement on what I am now. I incorporate my Vision that I see myself as a 180-pound fit man and I base my "I am" statement on my Vision.

What I gain from the "I am" statement is the understanding of what "I deserve." The second part of the Value Statement is where I think about and meditate on the benefits enjoyed by someone who is what I desire to be. I think about the benefits of being a healthy/fit 180-pound man. I deserve to be desired sexually by my wife. I deserve to spend time participating in activities with my children and grandchildren. I deserve to stay active and choose to eat healthy foods. I deserve to participate in 5Ks, 10Ks, and marathons.

I can apply the "I deserve" section to my Vision of myself as a Christian, a godly husband, an excellent employee or business owner, an excellent minister, a godly father, a financially wealthy man, etc. This is really a section to identify the dreams I have of what being healthy, wealthy, and wise looks and feels like. The dreams come with a cost. There is something I am obligated to do to realize my vision and dreams. For example, when I think about what I deserve as a 180-pound healthy man, I deserve to sleep without snoring; I deserve to breathe easily when I walk up a flight of stairs; I deserve to play with my children's children; I deserve to bless my wife sexually.

The last part of the Value Statement is where I acknowledge my obligations. To become a 180-pound fit man. I am obligated to pray for strength and discipline. I am obligated to increase my physical activity, (for example, I started walking and increasing my step goal from 5K to 10K to 11K to 15K to 20K per day). I am obligated to eat healthful foods. I am obligated to eat smaller portions. I am obligated to discipline my body. I am obligated to reduce the amount of sugar I eat. I am obligated to consistently maintain my healthy lifestyle.

Actions speak louder than words.
My actions (verb) will reflect my values (noun).

Chapter Review

Take a few minutes and review the **Ask Yourself** questions and the **Key Points** highlighted in this chapter.

Ask Yourself...
How do I show that I value my life, my God-given purpose, and God?

Ask Yourself...
What are my high-level values?
What are my low-level values?

Key Points Review:

> ➤ **Caleb valued his life, his purpose, and God.**

➢ **Actions speak louder than words. My actions (verb) will reflect my values (noun).**

Create your Value Statement using this format:

I am _____, I deserve _____, and I am obligated to _____.

Pray and ask God to forgive you when you have not put action behind what you say you value. Ask Him to show you the areas you need to begin to work on to improve your actions so they will reflect the value you place on your God-given vision.

CHAPTER 4

VOICE

NOW THAT I HAVE A VISION OF WHAT I WILL BECOME and I Value my Vision, I must learn to master the Voice of a **Victor**. Again, Caleb provides an excellent example of the power of the voice. The voice is not just what we say, but equally as important, what we hear and listen to. We all have an inner voice that speaks to us and through us. That voice charts the course of our lives.

Caleb especially had to deal with the "inner" voice, because he was surrounded by people amplifying their voices daily. As if his neighbors were in cahoots with the devil, they were constantly saying, "Hey Caleb, we'll never make it, I just know we won't!" I believe Caleb demonstrated how to silence that inner voice of doubt and fear and even negative words spoken by neighbors, friends, and loved ones. He spoke the word that Moses, the Man of God, spoke to him. He spoke that word for over forty years.

Ask Yourself…
Do I find myself speaking words of doubt and fear?

Do I repeat the negative words spoken by neighbors, friends, and even loved ones?

Voices of a Victor

As a noun, the definition of voice is the sound produced by the vocal organs of a vertebrate, especially a human; the ability to produce such sounds; the mind as it produces verbal thoughts; the distinctive style or manner of expression of an author or of a character in a book. As a verb, it means to express in words; utter.[6]

Reading these definitions, I realized I needed to listen to God's truth and stop listening to the lies of the devil. I needed to stop listening to my own negative self-defeating thoughts. I needed to stop listening to the culture's doom and gloom being spoken all around me. Instead, I had to learn to listen to the Voices of a **Victor**.

Ask Yourself...

Am I listening to God's truth or the lies of the devil?

Is my self-talk self-defeating?

Am I listening to the voices of doom and gloom all around me?

How is this affecting my journey from victim to victor?

Voices of a Victor

It just makes sense that if you want to learn how to do something, you find someone who is good at it or is an expert at that thing. Since God is the ultimate **Victor** and His wisdom on how to talk like a **Victor** is free, I decided to start with Him. The good thing is God still speaks today. He speaks through His Word. He speaks through His Holy Spirit. He speaks through angels. He speaks through other people. I am not telling you that I am God's press secretary, but as you read this book, God is speaking through me to you.

God desires and yearns to speak to us and through us today.

God speaks through His Word, so let's look at a couple of scriptures. First, "My sheep hear my voice, and I know them, and they follow me" (John 10:27 NKJV). How does this work? I will give you an example. One day in early May of 2015, I got on the treadmill and walked for 65 minutes. The display showed that I had burned 1352 calories. I was so excited! I thought, "Wow! I just burned a third of a pound in one workout!"

The enemy started laughing and said, "Ha! A third of a pound? A third of a pound? You need to lose 300 pounds and you are excited about a third of a pound? You ain't never gonna lose that weight, just quit!" Immediately, before discouragement could even try to set up camp, the Holy Spirit said, "And in 300 days you will have lost 100 pounds, KEEP GOING!"

Glory to God! I started crying because that "spirit of quitting" was broken! I chose to listen to the Holy Spirit and I kept praying, eating better, and walking. I lost 100 pounds in 320 days! Praise God! I am learning to filter out the voices of discouragement, doubt, and defeat.

Ask Yourself…

Am I listening to the voice of the Lord or the voice of the enemy?

Am I learning to filter out the voices of discouragement, doubt, and defeat?

In Mark 4:24, Jesus warns us, "Be diligent to understand the meaning behind everything you hear, for as you do, more understanding will be given to you. And according to the depth of your longing to understand, much more will be added to you" (TPT).[7] When I listen to network/cable news, watch the majority of TV/cable shows/programs, or R-rated or worse shows, it's like spiritual junk food.

**The key to my transformation came from the inside out.
True change happened spiritually.**

I changed my spiritual diet and soon I was able to change my physical diet. At first, I tried to accomplish this in my own strength and will power (mostly "won't" power). I would lose weight until I felt I had done good and should reward myself. Most of you know the routine. Back came the pounds and the fat and the guilt and the eating and the weight and so on. You get the picture.

I had to build up my spirit man so that it ruled my body/flesh. I believe that hearing and obeying the Holy Spirit's voice is what is helping me change. I make daily Bible reading, daily prayer, daily praying in other tongues, listening to biblical teaching throughout the day, and journaling my priorities. My spiritual nutrition is more important to me than my bodily nutrition. When I hear the Holy Spirit tell me that I do not need to eat a bowl of ice cream and I listen, I actually benefit bodily. The Holy Spirit prompted me to stop adding salt to my food. Prior to losing over 60 pounds, when I would get my blood pressure taken, the nurses would check it two or three times and then ask me if I had just come from working out. They would get the extended cuff, but it was still around 135 over 90-95.

When I was still about 70 pounds from my weight goal, I took a health risk assessment in February of 2017 and my blood pressure was 120/78. In fact, on that assessment, my cholesterol results were considered very good to near optimal, Look at what the Lord has done!

Listening to the Voice of God has paid off big time.

The Holy Spirit prompted me to start walking in place at work and now I walk at least 15K steps per day. The Holy Spirit advises me on how to respond to my wife and my children.

Huge benefits. Fellas, listen to God, He created her, formed her in the womb. Listen to God, Father knows best!

The enemy will constantly speak to you as well. The Bible records that he tempted Jesus, so you know he is going to come after us. The good thing is you can quickly recognize his voice when you hear words of discouragement like: "you're not good enough; you're too this or too that; you'll never be, or get, or have…" The enemy also speaks words of fear like: "you'll die if you…; you're going to fail; you'll go bankrupt; they hate you!" When you hear reminders of your past failures, you can be sure it's the devil. God tells us His plans for us are good, not evil.

**So, reject the voice of the devil.
Jesus tells us that His sheep will not follow the voice of
a stranger.**

Self-Talk

We also need to become aware of our own negative self-talk. We can be creatures of habit. For years, I laughed and joked about being the "Fat-cat from Alley-rats." I talked about how I could just smell a cake and gain 10 pounds. I called myself "Big Bob" and made jokes about my fatness. I would replay my failures and say, "I doubt it," "I don't know," "I could never do that," "It never fails." I was an addict to negative self-talk. It was so natural that it seemed like it was in me in abundance. I had to break that addiction.

Ask Yourself...

Am I addicted to negative self-talk?

In Matthew 12:34, Jesus explained that we will say with our mouths what is in our hearts in abundance. So, for me to change what I was saying I had to change what was in my heart. I made putting God's Word in my heart a priority. For years, I really wanted to lose weight, I really wanted to do better, I really wanted to improve. I would compromise when I really wanted to do something. I wouldn't stick with it and I wouldn't accomplish it.

Putting God's Word in your heart in abundance requires two things:

➤ **Feed on the Word** - Read the Bible, listen to biblical teachings, read books about becoming more Christ-like, pray constantly, and listen for God's voice.

➤ **Stop** putting anything else in your heart.

If an athlete trains to win the gold medal in the Olympics, and cuts out partying, eating junk food, and staying up late playing video games, we applaud them. We should applaud them because they have made the necessary sacrifices to achieve their goal. I believe getting God's Word in my heart in abundance is exactly the same. I am after a gold medal prize to be a **Victor!**

Ask Yourself…

As I think about my goal/objective/desire, do I believe such a sacrifice is really necessary?

The key is believing and saying what you really believe in your heart.

So, did I just start saying, "I'm a 180-pound fit man," and the next day I was 180 pounds? No! It was not even a year later. However, the more I said, "I am getting down to 180 pounds," the more I start to resemble that remark. The Bible says that we **will** have whatever we believe in our hearts and say. That's why just saying, "I'm a millionaire!" seldom works. You say that hoping one day you will hit the lottery or God will hear your confession and drop a little payment from Heaven in your backyard. Hoping for it doesn't mean you believe it, so you won't receive it.

I do believe that I am going to be a 180-pound fit man, so I say, "I am getting down to 180 pounds." I believe that even when I would step on the scale and my weight went up from the previous week. The more I say, "I am a **Victor not** a Victim," the more victories I experience in my life. My marriage is the best it has ever been. My children are pursuing a relationship with Jesus. My finances are getting better. My fear of failure is disappearing.

Romans chapter 8 is one of my favorite scripture passages. Romans 8:37 in particular says that we are more than conquerors through Him Who loved us. I am more than a conqueror! Hebrews 4:12 was another Scripture I had to speak over myself consistently. "For the Word that God speaks is alive and full of power [making it active, operative, energizing, and effective]..." (AMP).

I started saying, "I have God's Word in me, so I am Active, Operative, Energizing, and Effective!" When I first started saying that I felt like I was anything but active or effective. However, I kept saying it and I would come home and do stuff. I helped with the dishes, the laundry, change lightbulbs, collected the trash, etc. I started having managers at work tell me that they were looking to promote me. We were asked to help more on the marriage ministry team. I created a curriculum for our Men's Ministry Basic Training class. I began to become what I was speaking forth.

Chapter Review

So, to review this section on The **V**'s of being a **Victor**:

V - Get a **V**ision of who you really are and who you want to be.

V - Understand your **V**alue and determine what you **V**alue.

V - Then guard your heart so that you can hear the right **V**oice and give **V**oice to who you are and what you desire.

Ask Yourself...
  Do I find myself speaking words of doubt and fear?

Do I repeat the negative words spoken by neighbors, friends, and even loved ones?

Is this how I want to continue?

Ask Yourself...

Am I listening to God's truth or the lies of the devil?

Is my self-talk self-defeating?

Am I listening to the voices of doom and gloom all around me?

How is this affecting my journey from victim to victor?

Ask Yourself...

Am I listening to the voice of the Lord or the voice of the enemy?

Am I learning to filter out the voices of discouragement, doubt, and defeat?

Ask Yourself...

Am I addicted to negative self-talk?

Ask Yourself...

As I think about my goal/objective/desire, do I believe such a sacrifice is really necessary?

Key Points Review:

➢ **God desires and yearns to speak to us and through us today.**

➢ **The key to my transformation came from the inside out.**

➤ True change happened spiritually.

➤ Listening to the Voice of God has paid off big time.

➤ Reject the voice of the devil.

➤ Jesus tells us that His sheep will not follow the voice of a stranger.

➤ The key is believing and speaking what you really believe in your heart.

Positive Self-Talk begins by putting God's Word in your heart in abundance.

➤ **Feed on the Word** - Read the Bible, listen to biblical teachings, read books about becoming more Christ-like, pray constantly, and listen for God's voice.

➤ **Stop** putting anything else in your heart.

Record what God reveals to you from each of these scriptures:

John 10:27

Romans 8:37

Hebrews 4:12

Matthew 12:34

Mark 4:24

Pray and ask God to show you how to implement all of the principles presented in this section of moving from **Victim** to **Victor.**

PART 2

I

Chapter 5 - Identity
Chapter 6 - Integrity
Chapter 7 - Intelligence

Now that we have discussed the "V's" of being a Victor, let's move on to the "I's." All in favor say "I." The I's have it: Identity, Integrity, and Intelligence (Wisdom). In the Bible, Daniel is an excellent example that every Victor must know their true Identity, operate in complete Integrity, and constantly seek Intelligence (Wisdom). Let's start with Identity.

CHAPTER 5

IDENTITY

Who am I?

Why am I here?

What is my purpose?

Should I be doing that or should I be doing what they are doing?

Why am I so frustrated?

Why do I seem so lost, so out of place, so alone?

Who AM I?

I KNOW THESE ARE QUESTIONS THAT HAUNT MANY people. They have haunted me. I wanted to be liked, so I tried to fit in and be somebody that people liked. That last phrase is so filled with irony. Most of my life, my clothes were too tight. I looked like I was stuffed into them or bulging out of them. WOW! What a revelation. Inside, I also felt like I was squeezing into careers or relationships or ministry or life. I was bulging out of them and it was uncomfortable, even painful.

Outwardly, I was squeezing into clothes and bulging out of them and it was uncomfortable and painful. I thought I needed a different body to be a body shape that people liked. I tried to fit in and be some-BODY, any-BODY but this body! I feel like I just had a Bishop TD Jakes moment. Man, that is powerful! As I typed that, it just, BAM! hit me! Glory!

Ask Yourself…

Have I ever asked myself, "Who am I? What is my purpose?"

A dictionary definition of identity is, "the condition of being oneself or itself, and not another; condition or character as to who a person or what a thing is; the qualities, beliefs, etc., that distinguish or identify a person or thing; the sense of self, providing sameness and continuity in personality over time."[8]

I want to explain the difference between having a vision of who you are and knowing your identity. Your vision is typically who you want to be. You work toward reaching your vision. Your identity is who you are. The definition above says it is the condition of being oneself and not another.

As a Victim, I believed the qualities of fat/obesity, laziness, mediocrity, and failure were my distinguishing characteristics. I was fat, people enjoyed me as big Bob, big guy, big old Bob, etc. I liked not doing much, chillin', watching TV, etc. I was comfortable just keeping a job, watching over-achievers do "all that extra unnecessary stuff" and get promoted. I identified with the average Joe. Thank God, the Victor in me knew I had a true identity from God and I had to find out who I was.

One of the first things that stands out about Daniel is that when he was taken captive as a young man, his name was changed. Daniel was given a new identity. His captors placed a slave name on him, Belteshazzar. Maybe, because it was much harder to say than Daniel.

> *The chief official gave them new names: to Daniel, the name Belteshazzar; to Hananiah, Shadrach; to Mishael, Meshach; and to Azariah, Abednego. But Daniel resolved not to defile himself with the royal food and wine, and he asked the chief official for permission not to defile himself this way.*
> (Daniel 1:7-8)

I like verse 8 where it says, "Daniel resolved not to defile himself…this way." Daniel did not accept his slave name and he did not accept what the culture around him said was right. Daniel knew his identity and because of that, he refused to defile himself. That's what knowing your identity does for you. It is what knowing my identity did for me. I am a born-again child of God, I am a new creature in Christ, I am more than a conqueror. So, I started to realize that a child of God is not addicted to anything but God, the Word of God, His presence, and His Holy Spirit.

When we read the book of Daniel, he is referred to as Daniel. A few times, it is noted that he was called Belteshazzar, but a decade later King Darius calls him Daniel. I had to stop identifying with the labels I had been given by me and others. To be a Victor, I must identify with being a 180-pound healthy man as well as an abundantly wealthy man able to give to every good work and charitable donation. I will identify with being a loving, faithful, and dedicated husband, as well as a loving, fun, available father. I also identify with being a faithful, excellent ministry leader. Knowing my identity helps me make the right choices, I will discuss choices later.

A child of God loves people not food.
A child of God is active, not lazy.
A child of God makes a promise/commitment and keeps it.
A child of God is a Victor.
A Victor wins. A Victor overcomes. A Victor never quits!

The Bible has so much to say about who we truly are when we get born again. I like to read a book by Kenneth E. Hagin, "In Him." Rev. Hagin lists several scriptures that tell us who we are in Jesus, by Jesus, through Jesus, and because of Jesus. One of my favorites is, "Yet in all these things we are more than conquerors through Him who loved us" (Romans 8:37). The main point is I recognized that I am not a Victim, I am a Victor! I was made a new creation in Christ. I am who God says I am! I have what God says I have! I can do what God says I can do! I will give you a homework assignment below to find out what the Bible says about who you are in Christ.

Chapter Review

I suggest you take a few minutes and review the **Ask Yourself** questions and the **Key Points** highlighted in this chapter. Also, take the time to read and meditate on the **scriptures** that helped me on my journey from **Victim** to **Victor**.

Ask Yourself...
> *Who am I?*
> *Why am I here?*
> *What is my purpose?*
> *Should I be doing that or should I be doing what they are doing?*
> *Why am I so frustrated?*
> *Why do I seem so lost, so out of place, so alone?*

Key Points Review:

> ➢ **A child of God loves people not food.**
> ➢ **A child of God is active, not lazy.**
> ➢ **A child of God makes a promise/commitment and keeps it.**
> ➢ **A child of God is a Victor.**
> ➢ **A Victor wins. A Victor overcomes. A Victor never quits!**

Ask Yourself…

Am I a child of God?

Record what God reveals to you about who He says you are from each of these scriptures:

Romans 8:37
Romans 8:16-17
Revelation 12:11
John 16:27
John 15:16
2 Corinthians 5:17
1 Corinthians 1:30
1 Peter 2:4

Now answer the final question posed at the beginning of this chapter:

Who AM I?

Pray and ask God to continually remind you of your **I**dentity through His eyes. Pray and ask Him to open the eyes of your spirit to see you as He sees you. Declare this truth as you go through your day.

CHAPTER 6

INTEGRITY

THE NEXT I FACTOR IS INTEGRITY. NOW THAT I KNOW and believe who I truly am, I want to behave in accordance with my identity. A definition of integrity is, "the quality of being honest and having strong moral principles; moral uprightness; undivided; the state of being whole, entire, or undiminished; a sound, unimpaired, or perfect condition."[9]

The integrity of Daniel can best be confirmed by the Word of the Lord the prophet Ezekiel received in Ezekiel 14:12-23, the short version is: God identifies three men He considers full of integrity, Noah, Job, and Daniel. The Lord says that if a country sins against Him and He decides to destroy it, even if those three men lived in that country, they are the only three that would survive because of their integrity. Daniel also has the honor of being one of the few men in the Bible that has nothing bad said about him. In fact, his accusers had to make it against the law to obey God. That's integrity!

A major aspect of integrity is the quality of being honest.

Honest with whom, honest when, and honest where?

Honest with whom? I had to be honest with myself first. I, Bob Wells Jr., was voluntarily eating the wrong types of food and eating too much of it. I was sitting at work for 8-10 hours, and then coming home to sit and rest from a hard day of "work." I was doing a mediocre job at work by choice. I was not loving my wife as Christ loved the church. I was not living Jesus in front of my children, nor was I bringing them up in the fear and admonition of the Lord. I was my problem or the cause of my problems. I had to be honest with myself concerning becoming a 180-pound healthy man. I had to make better eating choices, I had to do more exercise, and I had to increase my actual exercise.

Ask Yourself...

Have I been being honest with myself about the true cause of my problems?

Honest when? The definition of integrity included having strong moral principles and moral uprightness. What does that have to do with being a Victor? Strong moral principles are a discipline. When I was a Cadet, we had a saying, "Choose to do the harder right versus the easier wrong." Because we had an honor code, it made it easier to follow that saying. It was still a choice and even with an honor code, I could sleep during the day instead of studying and be satisfied with the low grade that accompanied my poor decision. A Victim is always looking for the easy way out. Then when trouble arises a Victim cries about how they were tricked, or misled, or they never get a break, or wah, wah, wah. A Victor wants to win even if it means sacrifice, struggle, and extra effort! No more sweets/sugar, no excuses!

Ask Yourself...

Do I "choose to do the harder right versus the easier wrong"?

Do my choices reflect strong moral principles and moral uprightness?

Honest where? Integrity is also the state of being whole, entire, undivided, or undiminished. Here is where I have to take the Bible's declaration of our identity and accept it. I do not add to it or subtract from it. Integrity helps me stay completely the Righteousness of God in Christ Jesus. I read that, but I sin. I might use profanity, I might look at pornography, I might get drunk, I might steal time from my employer, I might forget to read my Bible, etc. So, there is no way I am righteous. Well, one of us is a liar. Either I'm lying or God, through His Word, is lying. The Word does **not** say if I never sin or always perform perfectly, then I might be as righteous as Jesus.

The Word says I AM the Righteousness
of God IN Christ Jesus
(2 Corinthians 5:21).

That settles it. Now, by faith, I trust God to consider me just as completely Righteous as He considers Jesus. By the way, I capitalize Righteous in some cases to emphasize that Righteousness is Jesus. So, I am still learning to trust that my identity in God's eyes is completely settled. I cannot add to it or subtract from it. Glory!

Chapter Review

I suggest you take a few minutes and review the **Ask Yourself** questions and the **Key Points** highlighted in this chapter. Also, take the time to read and meditate on the **scriptures** that helped me on my journey from **Victim** to **Victor**.

Ask Yourself...

Have I been being honest with myself about the true cause of my problems?

Ask Yourself...

Do I "choose to do the harder right versus the easier wrong"?

Do my choices reflect strong moral principles and moral uprightness?

Ask Yourself...

Whom am I to be honest with?

When am I to be honest?

Where am I to be honest?

Which of these areas do I need to work on?

Key Points Review:

> ➢ **A major aspect of integrity is the quality of being honest.**
> ➢ **"Choose to do the harder right versus the easier wrong."**
> ➢ **The Word says I AM the Righteousness of God IN Christ Jesus (2 Corinthians 5:21).**

Record what God reveals to you from each of these scriptures:

Ezekiel 14:12-23
2 Corinthians 5:21
2 Corinthians 5:20

Pray and ask God to continually show you how to represent Him with integrity as His ambassador to those in your area of influence.

CHAPTER 7

INTELLIGENCE
(WISDOM)

INTELLIGENCE IS CRUCIAL FOR A VICTOR. I AM USING
intelligence as a synonym for wisdom simply because Victor is
spelled with an "I" and is not spelled with a "W." The prophet
Ezekiel provides another Word from God about Daniel. This
time we read about his wisdom in Ezekiel 28:1-3.

> *The word of the LORD came to me: "Son of man,
> say to the ruler of Tyre, 'This is what the Sovereign
> LORD says: "...But you are a mere mortal and not
> a god, though you think you are as wise as a god. Are
> you wiser than Daniel?"'*

Another report of the wisdom of Daniel is found in Daniel
1:17 and 20.

> *As for these four young men, God gave them knowl-
> edge and skill in all literature and wisdom; and
> Daniel had understanding in all visions and*

dreams…And in all matters of wisdom and under-standing about which the king examined them, he found them ten times better than all the magicians and astrologers who were in all his realm.

I will begin with the definitions of intelligence and wisdom. Intelligence is, "the ability to learn or understand or to deal with new or trying situations; reason; also: the skilled use of reason; the ability to apply knowledge to manipulate one's environment or to think abstractly as measured by objective criteria (such as tests); mental acuteness; shrewdness; the act of understanding; comprehension; information concerning an enemy or possible enemy or an area."[10]

Wisdom is, "knowledge that is gained by having many experiences in life; the natural ability to understand things that most other people cannot understand; knowledge of what is proper or reasonable; good sense or judgment."[11]

Intelligence and wisdom go together like bread and butter. Each food can exist without the other. Some eat one without the other but adding butter to the bread makes the bread tastier and may even compensate for the plainness of the bread. Sometimes, intelligence can be dry, burnt, or old and stale. Wisdom comes along and we see the benefit of the intelligence or how to apply the intelligence. So, as the Bible tells us in Proverbs 4:7, "Wisdom is the principal thing; therefore get wisdom: and with all thy getting get understanding."

Wisdom = Knowledge + Understanding

Practically speaking, intelligence about any subject is readily available on the internet. I can do a search of any topic and get several hundred even thousands of results to look at. So, the knowledge about most topics is mine for the asking. Being willing or diligent to ask for it is another subject. Many times, I have been stubborn or prideful and just refused to seek the knowledge. I know it is out there, but I have decided that I will continue to operate in my own limited knowledge and try to force success to come to me. INSANITY! I know it's foolish, but stubbornness and pride ruled my thinking and actions and I continued to suffer defeat.

Albert Einstein said, "Insanity is doing the same thing, over and over again, but expecting different results."[12]

Ask Yourself...

Have I been repeating the same behavior but expecting different results?

How has that worked out for me?

You know the story. I wonder out loud why nothing is changing and why God doesn't help me or bless me or send a miracle, etc. Praise God, He is not a "stubborn, I'll show them, I told you so," Father. No, He is a loving patient Father.

Wisdom shouts in the street, She lifts her voice in the square; At the head of the noisy streets she cries out; At the entrance of the gates in the city she utters her sayings: "How long, O naive ones, will you love being simple-minded? And scoffers delight themselves in scoffing and fools hate knowledge? Turn to my reproof, behold, I will pour out my spirit on you; I will make my words known to you." (Proverbs 1:20-23)

So, I need to get over myself. I don't know it all, in fact, I have a lot to learn. So, the more I learn, the more victorious I become.

Ask Yourself…

Am I willing and diligent to seek knowledge?

Or have I been stubborn or prideful and just refused to seek the knowledge I need to be successful?

Specifically pertaining to weight loss and health, I had to seek knowledge about the basics of weight loss. I know this is going to sound too simple, but losing weight is a simple equation.

Consistent Calories Out (burned) > Calories In (eaten) = Weight Loss.

I tried eating less one day and weighing myself and I had gained a pound. So, "wisdom" makes the decision to **consistently** burn more calories than I eat. Now, I **know** that if I consistently burn more calories than I eat, I will lose weight. So, initially, I started walking and I was burning more calories than I had previously burned. However, I was still eating 2-3 slices of pizza, breakfast tacos, enchiladas, fried chicken, double cheeseburgers, and fries. Well, the scale still said, "One at a time, PLEASE!"

So, I'm walking 20-30 minutes per day 2-3 days per week, but I am gaining weight. What is the problem? I had to get **intelligence** on the calories in. So, I know it is a pain in the butt, but I found out that a slice of pizza can range from 400-1000 calories. That means one slice of deep-dish, meat-lovers, supreme-loaded pizza could wipe out 45-60 minutes of walking. Hello! I didn't know that. A cheeseburger combo meal could wipe out 45-60 minutes of walking. I decided to pay attention to how many calories I eat daily.

Wisdom kicked in. I also discovered that some calories are better than others. For instance, grilled chicken versus fried chicken. A four-ounce serving of grilled chicken breast is 180 calories and a four-ounce serving of fried chicken breast is 370 calories. So, I have never been able to eat half of a fried chicken breast. In addition, most people get sides like mashed potatoes with gravy or french fries, a biscuit, and a diet drink. I used to joke that the diet drink would absorb the other calories and fat. It didn't, but boy was it funny to say.

Anyway, back to wisdom and intelligence. Because our simple equation is not changing, but remains constant and consistent, by tracking the calories I was taking in, I found out that while I thought I was eating well, my calories-in were higher than my calories-out. By tracking my calories-in, I quickly realized that a handful of peanuts is a couple of hundred calories. So, I gathered intelligence about calories-in.

I use an app on my phone and search for the food I plan to eat or have eaten. The app gives me a selection of possible matches and I can get a good idea of how many calories I am eating. I use a fitness tracker to help me calculate how many calories I have burned. I know it sounds tedious and it's true I must discipline myself to do it. However, I now enjoy disciplining myself to track my calories. When I don't track my calories, it is easy to overeat and to make unhealthful food choices. Since I want to lose 180 pounds, I will track my calories.

Chapter Review

I suggest you take a few minutes and review the **Ask Yourself** questions and the **Key Points** highlighted in this chapter. Also, take the time to read and meditate on the **scriptures** that helped me on my journey from **Victim** to **Victor**.

Ask Yourself...

Have I been repeating the same behavior but expecting different results?

How has that worked out for me?

Ask Yourself...

Am I willing and diligent to seek knowledge?

Or have I been stubborn or prideful and just refused to seek the knowledge I need to be successful?

Key Points Review:

> ➤ **Wisdom = Knowledge + Understanding**
> ➤ **Albert Einstein said, "Insanity is doing the same thing, over and over again, but expecting different results."[13]**

Record what God reveals to you from each of these scriptures:

Ezekiel 28:1-3

Daniel 1:17-20

Proverbs 4:7

Proverbs 1:20-23

Pray and ask God to show you how to effectively implement Proverbs 4:7 in your life. Consistently seek knowledge and understanding so you can make intelligent choices and continually move from **Victim** to **Victor**.

PART 3

C

We are cruising along, we have passed through the **V**'s and the **I**'s, next stop the **C**'s. In the **C**'s, I had to learn the importance of **my** choices, get serious about my **C**ommitment and **C**onsistency, and build up my **C**ourage. I learned these lessons by studying the book of Nehemiah. Let's keep cruising.

CHAPTER 8

CHOICES

GO OUT TO EAT OR ORDER PIZZA? GO TO A MOVIE OR stream several at home? Tex-Mex or BBQ? Italian or Chinese? Which Shirt? What pants? Finish writing the book or watch a movie? **Choices!** We are constantly faced with choices. Most of our choices are the mundane ordinary choices I listed above. The Bible character I want to study concerning Choices, Commitment/ Consistency, and Courage is Nehemiah. Nehemiah faced situations and circumstances that had significant consequences attached to his Choices, Commitment, and Courage.

In the book of Nehemiah, we see one of the first choices he needs to make is whether to keep his important, secure, comfortable government job or choose to risk it to help his people in Jerusalem.

"And it came to pass in the month of Nisan, in the twentieth year of King Artaxerxes, when wine was before him, that I took the wine and gave it to the king. Now I had never been sad in his presence

before. Therefore the king said to me, "Why is your face sad, since you are not sick? This is nothing but sorrow of heart." So I became dreadfully afraid, and said to the king, "May the king live forever! Why should my face not be sad, when the city, the place of my fathers' tombs, lies waste, and its gates are burned with fire?" Then the king said to me, "What do you request?" So I prayed to the God of heaven. And I said to the king, "If it pleases the king, and if your servant has found favor in your sight, I ask that you send me to Judah, to the city of my fathers' tombs, that I may rebuild it." Then the king said to me (the queen also sitting beside him), "How long will your journey be? And when will you return?" So it pleased the king to send me; and I set him a time." (Nehemiah 2:1-6 NKJV)

Nehemiah heard a report that Jerusalem and the people living there were in tough times. Nehemiah could have chosen to say, "I'll pray for them." Or say, "If they need anything, let me know." There is nothing wrong with praying or offering to help. However, choosing to leave your comfort zone, risking your life and livelihood, rolling up your sleeves and getting dirty is taking it to the next level.

Like Nehemiah, I have discovered that my life is a result of the choices I have made.

Those choices fall under one of two headings: Life or Death. In Deuteronomy 30:19-20, Moses said, "I call heaven and earth to witness this day against you that I have set before you life and death, the blessings and the curses; therefore choose life, that you and your descendants may live, and may love the Lord your God, obey His voice, and cling to Him. For He is your life and the length of your days, that you may dwell in the land which the Lord swore to give to your fathers, to Abraham, Isaac, and Jacob" (ESV).

In Proverbs 18:21, God tells us that what we say is a key to choosing Life or Death. Also, in Romans 8:1-3, Paul tells us that our faith in Jesus gives us access to the Spirit of Life and frees us from the Spirit of Sin and Death.

The definition of Choice is: The act of choosing; the act of picking or deciding between two or more possibilities; the opportunity or power to choose between two or more possibilities; the opportunity or power to make a decision; a range of things that can be chosen.[14] So, as I live a life of a Victor, I have to recognize that every day, sometimes every minute of every day, I am offered a Choice between Life and Death.

I can choose to eat bacon and eggs, pancakes with syrup and whipped cream, hash browns, and buttermilk biscuits with gravy, or I can choose an egg white vegetable omelet with reduced salt added and two turkey sausages and eat until I am full. One choice leads to Death the other choice leads to Life.

I can choose to sit for hours watching TV, particularly, men that are fit and do a strenuous sport or I can get up and walk or do pushups or crunches, or **something**! Either way, it's **my** Choice. Since I have started choosing to eat healthful foods and exercise, I have lost over 100 pounds and I have kept it off. I like being able to breathe normally after climbing a flight of stairs or two. I like being able to stop eating when I am full. I like being able to stay awake when people are talking to me. I like being able to see some of the "V" shape coming in instead of the round or block shape. It starts with a Choice.

Ask Yourself...

What choices do I have that ultimately lead to Life or Death?

I had to get wisdom on some things in order to choose Life. For instance, I learned the best foods for me to eat. I do better not eating breads, starches (like mashed potatoes, rice, pastas, etc.), and sugars (like cookies, cakes/pies, donuts, candy bars, etc.). When I eat lean meats like chicken, turkey, fish, 90 percent lean hamburger, my body processes these foods better and faster. I can drink 100+ ounces of water per day. I can eat an apple instead of an apple pie or an apple fritter. The point is, I did the research to determine what is best for my body. You need to do the same thing.

I had to learn about "metabolism." Metabolism is how efficiently my body processes the food I eat. I learned that the faster my metabolism, the faster I burn calories. I learned that some foods drastically slow down my metabolism, like fried foods, highly processed foods, starches, and sugars from pies, cakes, candy bars, etc. I am sure that 99.99 percent of people will have the same results when it comes to fried foods, starches, sugars, etc. Sitting around or long periods of inactivity will also slow down my metabolism.

Once you know which foods bring Life and which lead to Death, you get to make the Choice. If you choose death, understand that you can do exercise to help fight the Death effects, but typically those foods make you not want to exercise. Really, the more I think about it, the foods that are better for you give you the energy to want to exercise.

Funny how a Choice for Death leads to more death and a Choice for life leads to more life.

Knowing what exercises are best for you requires wisdom as well. I walked, and I continue to walk. I enjoy walking. I put my headphones on and listen to Praise and Worship, Kenneth Copeland, Kenneth Hagin, Joseph Prince, Archie Neal, and Creflo A. Dollar Jr. to name a few. I started adding weightlifting once I had lost over 100 pounds. Some people may need to go to a more extreme exercise like CrossFit training or something like that. The point is, find out what your body responds to best in combination with the correct eating plan, and you will see results.

Once you know what Life or Death for you is—Choose Life!

Chapter Review

I suggest you take a few minutes and review the **Ask Yourself** questions and the **Key Points** highlighted in this chapter. Also, take the time to read and meditate on the **scriptures** that helped me on my journey from Victim to Victor.

Ask Yourself...
What choices do I have that ultimately lead to Life or Death?

Key Points Review:

➢ **Funny how a Choice for Death leads to more death and a Choice for life leads to more life.**
➢ **Once you know what Life or Death for you is— Choose Life!**

Record what God reveals to you about who He says you are from each of these scriptures.

Nehemiah 2:1-6
Deuteronomy 30:19-20
Proverbs 18:21
Romans 8:1-3

CHAPTER 9

COMMITMENT/CONSISTENCY

THIS NEXT PRINCIPLE IS VITAL TO A LIFE AS A VICTOR—
Commitment and its wonder twin Consistency. For me, it is
difficult to talk of one without the other. It is hard to convince
me that I am committed to a purpose/cause/goal if I am not
consistent. Nehemiah's commitment to rebuilding the walls in
Jerusalem is evidenced by his consistency.

> *"So, I sent messengers to them, saying, 'I am doing a
> great work, so that I cannot come down. Why should
> the work cease while I leave it and go down to you?'
> But they sent me this message four times, and I
> answered them in the same manner... So the wall
> was finished on the twenty-fifth day of Elul, in fif-
> ty-two days. And it happened, when all our enemies
> heard of it, and all the nations around us saw these
> things, that they were very disheartened in their
> own eyes; for they perceived that this work was done
> by our God."* (Nehemiah 6:3-4, 15-16 NKJV)

Nehemiah was committed to the work, so even when the distractions came to draw him away, he was consistent to keep putting a brick on top of a brick and in fifty-two days the wall was built.

For me, losing weight is a great work. When I commit to losing weight, and I have the V's, the I's, and I know the Choices to make, then I will consistently make the right (life/victor) choices. I have voiced a commitment to lose weight and I make a choice to eat a veggie egg white omelet for breakfast, a salad with vinaigrette dressing, and a grilled chicken breast with broccoli for dinner, Yay me!

If I eat a veggie egg white omelet for breakfast, a double cheeseburger and large fries for lunch, and fried chicken with mashed potatoes and gravy for dinner, then I show am **not** committed to losing weight because I am not being consistent in changing my diet.

I work out or in my case walk for thirty minutes three days in a row and then it rains on the fourth day and it takes me two weeks to get back in the "routine" of walking. Laugh, I know I'm the only one, but that is why Commitment and Consistency are wonder twins.

Ask Yourself…

What have I committed to that I am consistent at?

What have I committed to that I have found myself not consistent at?

Alert! Bunny trail/meddling coming up! Married men, we say we are committed to loving our wives as Christ loved the church, and then she says/does/doesn't do/keeps doing something that offends us.

Ask Yourself...
What if Jesus responded to me the way I respond to my wife?

I don't even want to think about it. I have to consistently forgive, consistently proactively do things to show her I love her, consistently provide for her, and consistently pray for and with her. I think you get the picture.

An important key to being Consistent in your Commitment is reading the Word about God's faithfulness and consistency.

The Holy Spirit lives in believers and we are supposed to bear much fruit. To achieve this, you need to say to yourself that you are Committed and you will Consistently do, say, and be the victorious person God created you to be. More practically, you will have to go military on yourself. When I was developing a battle plan in my Army days, I would set up checkpoints that we had to reach by a certain time. If we were defending, I had a timeline to have patrols out setting up early warning, dig foxholes, put mines and tripwires in place, etc. My platoon had a final objective and we had minor objectives to accomplish to ensure we could get to the main objective.

So, set little goals, like make your bed before you leave home and wash your dish after you use it. Start setting goals in small mundane daily tasks and accomplish them. Then start setting goals to be consistent in bigger things like putting the toilet seat down or complimenting your spouse. Then move on to bigger tasks like walking 30 minutes every day, praying in the Spirit thirty minutes each day, reading through the Bible in a year, and eating fruit instead of cakes/pies/donuts, etc. Start with something small and easy and feel good about being consistent in a small thing. Then tackle a bigger thing and more big things. You can do it.

I would pray Philippians 2:13 and 4:13 like this: "Lord, I am willing to be willing. I know You are working in me the desire to do Your will and giving me the ability to do Your will, so I can do all things through Christ which gives me strength!"

Chapter Review

I suggest you take a few minutes and review the **Ask Yourself** questions and the **Key Points** highlighted in this chapter. Also, take the time to read and meditate on the **scriptures** that helped me on my journey from Victim to Victor.

Ask Yourself...

What have you committed to that you are consistent at?

What have you committed to that you have found yourself not consistent at?

Ask Yourself...
What if Jesus responded to me the way I respond to my wife?

Key Point Review:

➤ **An important key to being Consistent in your Commitment is reading the Word about God's faithfulness and consistency.**

Record what God reveals to you about who He says you are from each of these scriptures.

Nehemiah 6:3-4, 15-16
Philippians 2:13
Philippians 4:13

CHAPTER 10

COURAGE
(TAKE ACTION)

I LIKE QUOTING LINES FROM MOVIES. THINKING ABOUT Courage makes me think about the cowardly lion in the Wizard of Oz, "put 'em up, put 'em up!"

Thankfully, Nehemiah provides us with a better example of having Courage. When he asked King Artaxerxes to go to Jerusalem, that took courage. More than once he confronted the Jewish nobles and rulers about mistreating fellow Jews. Another one of my favorite Scripture passages is found in Nehemiah 4:14-17.

> *And I looked, and arose and said to the nobles, to the leaders, and to the rest of the people, "Do not be afraid of them. Remember the Lord, great and awesome, and fight for your brethren, your sons, your daughters, your wives, and your houses." And it happened, when our enemies heard that it was known to us, and that God had brought their plot to nothing, that all of us returned to the wall, everyone*

to his work. So it was, from that time on, that half of my servants worked at construction, while the other half held the spears, the shields, the bows, and wore armor; and the leaders were behind all the house of Judah. Those who built on the wall, and those who carried burdens, loaded themselves so that with one hand they worked at construction, and with the other held a weapon." (Nehemiah 4:14-17 NKJV)

I love how this says, "**Don't** be afraid of them! **Fight** for your children, wife, prosperity, health, dream, etc." With one hand they worked at construction and the other hand they held a weapon. So, for you and me that means we change our diets and get active on the natural side, and we pray while we are doing it. I prefer to pray in the Spirit because I know I am getting double for my efforts.

Courage means the ability to do something that frightens one; strength in the face of pain or grief. A few synonyms for courage are: bravery, valor, nerve, fearlessness, intrepidity, daring, audacity, boldness, grit, true grit, heroism, and gallantry.[15]

A Victor must have Courage to take action.
You must act to accomplish anything.

Very seldom does anyone walk up and say, "I know you have been sitting around waiting for the rewards for sitting around.

So, here you go. I am going to give you everything you desire. You just sit back and relax." In fact, that never happens. You and I have to do something to get results. So, starting to exercise or change your diet takes Courage.

However, fear and doubt are constant companions of victims. What if I...and bad thing happens? What if I... and I fail? What if I ask... and says "NO!"? What if I... and I die?

Ask Yourself...

Have I ever asked myself, "what if bad things happen, what if I fail, what if I am rejected, what if I die" to keep me from taking action?

Courage answers these questions and says go for it. Other people have failed and recovered. In fact, 99.9 percent of highly successful people have failed multiple times. As Pastor Rick says, "Fellas, ask her out! You already got 'no' working for you! The worst that happens is you end up just like you are!" Don't respond by saying, "I can't handle rejection!" Get some courage, get rejected a bunch of times, and realize everybody gets rejected. Again, 99.9 percent of successful people heard several "no's" before they heard a single "yes"!

Courage got them in that position. You and I have to have Courage. When it comes to losing weight, consider the seriousness of doing nothing. It's not just that you will die. Everybody is going to die! You will live a life of embarrassment, pain, health issues, being short of breath, dreading to try to fasten the seat belt on an airplane or needing an extension. You will be the brunt of jokes, some that you may even start yourself. You will miss out on living and enjoying doing things with your children/grandchildren. I am sure some overweight people are not bothered by those concerns, but I am.

I want to live the best life I possibly can. Battling diabetes, heart disease, knee and back pain, and injury are not the best life possible. I enjoy being active now. I enjoy eating foods that improve my health. I enjoy seeing my kids happy that I am taking care of myself. I enjoy my wife being attracted to me. I was not a man of action. I made excuses. I avoided hard work and diligence like they were fatal diseases. I wanted to lose weight and I knew I needed to exercise and eat healthier to lose weight.

I know it sounds like a cliché, but I had a "come to Jesus meeting." I cried out to the Lord and asked Him to help me get my butt in gear. I read scriptures like Joshua 1:6-9; Philippians 4:13, 2 Timothy 1:7, Romans 8:15, 37-39, and 1 John 4:4, 17-18. These scriptures helped me build up my Courage. Eventually, I had to take a step and literally started walking. I did not start trying to lose 180 pounds in one day. I set my mind to the reality that it would take one to two years to reach my goal. I am still working toward my goal. The point is, pray for the Courage to take the first step, read scriptures about Courage and about the people in the Bible who showed Courage, and then just get to steppin'!

Chapter Review

I suggest you take a few minutes and review the **Ask Yourself** questions and the **Key Points** highlighted in this chapter. Also, take the time to read and meditate on the **scriptures** that helped me on my journey from Victim to Victor.

Ask Yourself...

Have I ever asked myself, "what if bad things happen, what if I fail, what if I am rejected, what if I die" to keep me from taking action?

Key Points Review:

➢ **A Victor has to have Courage to take action.**
➢ **You have to take action to accomplish anything.**

Record what God reveals to you about who He says you are from each of these scriptures.

Nehemiah 4:14-17
Joshua 1:6-9
Philippians 4:13
2 Timothy 1:7
Romans 8:15, 37-39
1 John 4:4, 17-18.

PART 4

T

We are really cruising now, I have covered the "**V**," "**I**," & "**C**" of being a **V**ictor. Now let's cover the "**T**." A victor has and uses his **T**alent(s), **expects** and overcomes **T**est/**T**rials, and accepts that being a victor takes **T**ime. I looked at the life of Joseph as my biblical example for the **T**s of being a victor.

Chapter 11

Talent

Many Bible scholars have studied and written commentaries on Joseph. I just want to acknowledge that Joseph had many talents. Some of his talents were dreaming, interpreting dreams, observing, and reporting, along with leadership and management. I know daydreaming is a talent many people have, but Joseph was given dreams by God.

Now Joseph had a dream, and he told it to his brothers; and they hated him even more. So he said to them, "Please hear this dream which I have dreamed: There we were, binding sheaves in the field. Then behold, my sheaf arose and also stood upright; and indeed your sheaves stood all around and bowed down to my sheaf." And his brothers said to him, "Shall you indeed reign over us? Or shall you indeed have dominion over us?" So they hated him even more for his dreams and for his words. Then he dreamed still another dream and told it to his brothers, and said, "Look, I have dreamed another dream. And this time, the sun, the moon, and the eleven stars bowed down to me." So he told it to his father and his brothers; and his father rebuked him and said to him, "What is this dream that you have dreamed? Shall your mother and I and your brothers indeed come to bow down to the earth before you?" And his brothers envied him, but his father kept the matter in mind. (Genesis 37:5-11 NKJV)

Joseph also had the God-given ability to interpret dreams.

And they said to him, "We each have had a dream, and there is no interpreter of it." So Joseph said to them, "Do not interpretations belong to God? Tell them to me, please." Then the chief butler told his dream to Joseph, and said to him, "Behold, in my dream a vine was before me, and in the vine were three branches; it was as though it budded, its blossoms shot forth, and its clusters brought forth ripe grapes. Then Pharaoh's cup was in my hand; and I took the grapes and pressed them into Pharaoh's cup, and placed the cup in Pharaoh's hand." And Joseph said to him, "This is the interpretation of it: The three branches are three days. Now within three days Pharaoh will lift up your head and restore you to your place, and you will put Pharaoh's cup in his hand according to the former manner, when you were his butler....When the chief baker saw that the interpretation was good, he said to Joseph, "I also was in my dream, and there were three white baskets on my head. In the uppermost basket were all kinds of baked goods for Pharaoh, and the birds ate them out of the basket on my head." So Joseph answered and said, "This is the interpretation of it: The three baskets are three days. Within three days Pharaoh will lift off your head from you and hang you on a tree; and the birds will eat your flesh from you." Now it came to pass on the third day, which was Pharaoh's birthday, that he made a feast for all his servants; and he lifted up the head of the chief butler and of the chief baker among his servants. Then he restored the chief butler to his butlership again, and he placed the cup in Pharaoh's hand. But he hanged the chief baker, as Joseph had interpreted to them. (Genesis 40:8-22 NKJV)

I only expounded upon the dreams and interpreting them because those types of talents are not usually seen as financial/career talents, and I was/am guilty of overlooking a God-given talent because I don't see how I can make money with the talent.

Believing you have at least one talent and probably several talents is another key to the transformation from Victim to Victor.

A definition of Talent is a special often athletic, creative, or artistic aptitude; general intelligence or mental power; ability; the natural endowments of a person.[16] We all have at least one talent. I am a natural encourager. I love to encourage people. I can't help it. I just do it! For years, I did not think much of that gift/talent. I did not see the value in encouraging people. In fact, I remember when one of my bosses was leaving for another position and he told me that I had to be one of the nicest men he knew. I was offended. I thought he was putting me down. He was complimenting me, but I did not think being nice and encouraging people was a talent.

The Holy Spirit, primarily through my wife, helped me to see how valuable my talent is. Recently, I just did what I do and greeted a co-worker, with a big smile and a word of encouragement, "Jimmy! Today is your day, Jimmy! You can make a difference in someone's life today!" He said thanks and I went on my way. About thirty minutes later, he stopped by my desk as I was talking with a customer/member, and he waited for me to finish. Then he told me that he printed off an encouraging email I had sent him a couple of months earlier and that he looked at it when he was having a "blah" day.

Then he said, "Bob, you didn't know this, but today is my thirty-year anniversary with the company, and when you said that this morning it really meant a lot to me. I just wanted to thank you and let you know that you are one of those people that when others see you, our day brightens. You smile, you are positive, and you just make people feel better. Thank you!"

WOW! I was overwhelmed. I do it because I love doing it, not because I want someone to praise me. Hearing that my gift lifts people up, WOW!

Great Bob, you encourage people, nice, what does that have to do with being a Victor? I'm glad you asked. When you recognize you have a talent, begin to see how that talent adds value to others. Appreciate your talent, begin to cultivate and enhance your talent, and most importantly use your talent.

Ask Yourself...

Have I recognized one of my talents?
Do I see how this talent adds value to others?
Do I appreciate my talent?
How am I using my talent?

There is a saying that tells us "success breeds success." In fact, scientific studies have been conducted and confirmed that success does breed success. That's why you should make yourself make your bed every morning. If you have children, give them small easy to achieve tasks like make your bed, brush your teeth, be ready to go on time, etc. and reward them for each success.

So, when I started seeing how my talent to encourage people had a positive impact, I was inspired to succeed at losing weight. Most of us have more than one talent, so recognize how you succeed in several areas, and then apply that spirit of success to challenges that you have not or had not been able to defeat.

I am warning you that the enemy will attempt to discourage you. In fact, he has been working on discouraging you most of your life. You have had people tell you what you cannot do, what you should not do, and what you will never do. You have had close friends and family who remind you of past tries and failures. You have had people you respect and admire ignore you or your ideas. Now that you are deciding to be a victor and defeat a giant that has stepped in front of you, the enemy shouts, "Don't forget how many times you have failed! Don't forget you will never amount to anything! Don't forget you always screw up!"

That is why you must use your talent and log some successes. Seriously, if you are so overcome by the belief that you only have failures in your past, then start with small victories, like making your bed every day and reading Psalm 23:1 every day.

Start with small victories and build on them.

Chapter Review

I suggest you take a few minutes and review the **Ask Yourself** questions and the **Key Points** highlighted in this chapter. Also, take the time to read and meditate on the **scriptures** that helped me on my journey from Victim to Victor.

Ask Yourself…

Have I recognized one of my talents?
Do I see how this talent adds value to others?
Do I appreciate my talent?
How am I using my talent?

Key Points Review:

➢ **Believing you have at least one talent and probably several talents is another key to the transformation from Victim to Victor.**
➢ **Start with small victories and build on them.**

Record what God reveals to you about who He says you are from each of these scriptures.

Genesis 37:5-11
Genesis 40:8-22
Psalm 23:1

CHAPTER 12

TESTS/TRIALS

IT SHOULD NOT COME AS A SURPRISE THAT THE PRImary measurement of whether you are a victor or not is by being tested or tried. In fact, anything of value has to be verified or tested. A diamond is tested on the 4 "C's" —Cut, Color, Clarity, and Carat. If someone walked up to you and showed you a clear gem the size of a walnut and asked you to pay them $1 Million for it, assuming you had $1 Million, of course, you would have the gem tested before you paid anything. Likewise, just because I say, "I am a Victor!" does not mean I am a Victor. I may be on my way to being a Victor, but I must have at least one victory.

So, a Victor will have **T**ests/**T**rials that they pass/overcome. The definition of a test is a procedure intended to establish the quality, performance, or reliability of something, especially before it is taken into widespread use; an event or situation that reveals the strength or quality of someone or something by putting them under strain.[17]

By putting us under strain,
our strength or endurance is revealed.

I know many pastors and ministers have reminded us that when we are under strain, our strength and quality are being revealed! We don't want to whine and complain when we are under strain, we want to endure and go through the pain and get all kinds of gain. In the military, there is a phrase, "embrace the suck!" The phrase means, "yes, it sucks, so deal with it! Stop wasting time wallowing in self-pity and hourly 'why me?' sessions. Embrace the suck!"

I want to look at a definition of a trial as well. Trial is trouble or grief; an annoying or frustrating person or thing.[18] Trouble or grief can be caused by and often compounded by an annoying person or frustrating thing. You and I think we are being punished because of the nosey, lazy, obnoxious, or annoying co-worker. No, we are being given an opportunity to rise above the situation, to demonstrate love, forgiveness, understanding, and grace—to be a victor.

When you need $100 for groceries and gas, and then the A/C unit stops in July in Texas, a Victor has a different mindset. A victor sees the trials as a challenge that will be overcome and springs into a confident action saying, "I can do all things through Christ, who strengthens me!" A Victim falls into pitiful self-pity and defeat saying, "Why me? I never get a break! Nothing good ever happens to/for me!" I say it again, "Embrace the suck!"

Ask Yourself…

Do I see a trial or a test as a challenge to overcome?
Do I embrace the suck?

Joseph has so many examples of going through tests and trials. His brothers despised him. The Bible says they hated him. His brothers conspired to kill him but decided to just sell him into slavery instead. He was a slave, then he was accused of rape, and though he was innocent, he went to prison. While in prison, he interprets dreams for two other prisoners and asked them to help him. One gets beheaded as Joseph said he would, so of course, he couldn't help him, but the other guy forgets for a couple of years. Well, Joseph, is a victor and realizes God is with him during all the "suck" and he just excels. We know Joseph embraced the suck because when he meets up with his brothers again, he is the number two man in Egypt, and they are afraid he will kill them.

> *Joseph said to them, "Do not be afraid, for am I in the place of God? But as for you, you meant evil against me; but God meant it for good, in order to bring it about as it is this day, to save many people alive. Now therefore, do not be afraid; I will provide for you and your little ones."* (Genesis 50:19-21 NKJV)

He comforted them and spoke kindly to them. We can infer from what we read about Joseph that he had the right attitude as he went through each test and trial. He had dreams that his brothers and parents would bow down to him and he never lost that vision and it eventually happened, despite all the tests and trials.

To paraphrase what Jesus said in John 16:33, "Look, you are going to have some problems, just accept that problems are going to come your way. But get your mind right! Be confident you will overcome the problems because I already overcame everything this world can bring!"

We don't pray for tests/trials.
We face them knowing we will have the victory!

Chapter Review

I suggest you take a few minutes and review the **Ask Yourself** questions and the **Key Points** highlighted in this chapter. Also, take the time to read and meditate on the **scriptures** that helped me on my journey from **Victim** to **Victor**.

Ask Yourself...

Do I see a trial or a test as a challenge to overcome?
Do I embrace the suck?

Key Points Review:

> ➤ By putting us under strain, our strength or quality is revealed.
> ➤ We don't pray for tests/trials. We face them knowing we will have the victory!

Record what God reveals to you about who He says you are from each of these scriptures.

Genesis 50:19-21
John 16:33

CHAPTER 13

TIME

FINALLY! SOME GOOD NEWS, BEING A VICTOR HAP-
pens instantly! Actually, we make a quality decision and declare:
"Today, I decree and declare I am a Victor. I break all ties to
the Victim mentality that has kept me bound for years! **I am
a victor!**" Awesome! Continue to make that confession daily.
But, did you hear the bubble burst? You must go through some
stuff (tests/trials). You need to demonstrate you are victor consistently. This means Time is involved.

I really get excited when I read words like "suddenly, immediately, at that very moment, instantly, and it happened." Those
words are so sweet. However, I have learned that many of those
"suddenlies" happened after years of waiting and expecting. In
fact, God is waiting for a suddenly. In a moment, "in the twin-
kling of an eye, Jesus will descend with a shout, and those that
are asleep will rise first and we who are alive will meet Him
in the air" (1 Corinthians15:52). Hallelujah! In the meantime,
God is patiently working on, in, and through you and me to
get to His suddenly!

I know that one of the many first times I tried to lose weight by my own will power, I got on the treadmill and after 10 minutes and sweating profusely, I prayed, "God, I need a miracle, just take this weight off of me and I will exercise and eat right to keep it off. Just do a miracle and take this weight off!" God is so cool. He has a great sense of humor. He replied, "Bob, a big guy like you gets on the treadmill for 60 minutes and doesn't have a heart attack, that IS a miracle." I love the Lord. Well, I didn't want that miracle back then, so I quit exercising, I never got around to changing my diet, and I gained an additional 100 pounds.

When the Victor mentality kicked in, I welcomed the truth that I would have to put in the effort for some time, like until I die or Jesus comes back. I realized that being healthy, losing weight, and getting the fat off would take time. I was ready for and equal to the challenge. I used to think of losing weight as a temporary change in behavior. Then, I realized that it is a lifestyle change. So, now I am **not** looking forward to the time when I can eat pizza, fried chicken, apple pie with ice cream, etc. Instead, I want to eat foods that are good for me. I see myself eating grilled chicken or salmon with broccoli when I am ninety. I see myself doing 10Ks and marathons when I am ninety. I see myself being active and productive in my later years.

Ask Yourself…

Do I see myself maintaining a healthy lifestyle for the rest of my life?

*Am I committed to being a **Victor for Life?***

Recognizing that my goal is a healthy lifestyle for the rest of my life helps me embrace the time requirement. I am pleased that I have been improving for three years now. I look forward to being successful for five years, ten years, and twenty-five years.

The key to being committed to being a Victor for Life, is to be a Victor one day at a time.

I know that is so cliché, banal, trite, hackneyed, and overused. However, it is true! When I thought about losing 180 pounds, I wanted to lose about 179 pounds in a day and the last pound in a couple of days after that. However, I knew that was not going to happen and I certainly didn't believe it would. So, I set mental goals, like I can lose four pounds per week and in forty-five weeks I will hit my goal. To lose four pounds per week, I need to lose about ½ pound per day. However, I didn't lose four pounds per week, but I did lose 1-2 pounds per week. Knowing that it would take me forty-five weeks, and that is nearly a year, I didn't get discouraged and quit. I just kept pushing because as a Victor, I know I am going to get down to 180 pounds!

Joseph also knew it would take time. He had his dreams of his brothers and parents bowing down to him when he was a teenager. Then he was a slave and in prison for several years. In fact, we are told that it was two years after he interpreted the dream for his fellow prisoner before he was released from prison and "suddenly" became Pharaoh's second in charge. The Bible says he was twenty years old. Then Egypt enjoyed seven good years, then the famine hit, and his brothers came and bowed down to him.

I know Bob Wells Jr. would have been praying and asking God: *when are my brothers going to bow down to me while I was a slave, a prisoner.* The same day I was "suddenly" the #2 man in Egypt, I would have sent soldiers to go get them and drag them before me. Ah, but a victor understands time and timing, and most importantly, trusting God! I was listening to a teaching that was discussing "suddenly" moments. The minister referred to 2 Kings 7:1. I got so excited because I love "suddenlies"! Elisha told the king and all the people that tomorrow the famine would be over. Hallelujah! So, I knew I wanted to meditate on that verse for the day.

I like to read and speak the same verse in the different versions of the Bible—NKJV, NIV, AMP, KJV, NLT, etc. So, as I read the verse in the International Children's Bible (ICB) which tells us Elisha said, "Listen to the Lord's word. This is what he says: 'About this time tomorrow 7 quarts of fine flour will be sold for two-fifths of an ounce of silver. And 13 quarts of barley will be sold for two-fifths of an ounce of silver. This will happen at the gate of Samaria.'"

In the New Century Version (NCV) it says Elisha said, "Listen to the Lord's word. This is what the Lord says: 'About this time tomorrow seven quarts of fine flour will be sold for two-fifths of an ounce of silver, and thirteen quarts of barley will be sold for two-fifths of an ounce of silver. This will happen at the gate of Samaria.'"

The Holy Spirit stopped me and had me read the first portion: "Listen to the Lord's Word. This is what the Lord says:_____. Then add the last part: "This will happen…" Glory to God! The Holy Spirit gave me a revelation that I have to listen to the Lord's Word, then find out what the Lord said. For example, "by His stripes I was healed, my God shall supply all my needs, I have no greater joy than hearing my children walk in truth, what God has joined together, let not man put asunder, I am the head and not the tail, the Lord is my Shepherd, I shall not want, etc." In His Word, we are assured that what the Lord says **will** happen! I shared that with my men's group and several other brothers, and they were immediately blessed.

The next evening, my air conditioner's blower motor stopped working. This time, instead of whining and complaining, I trusted God and He provided for us to stay with our in-laws and then to save money on the cost of repair. We learned to deal with a little discomfort while we waited for the suddenly financial blessing that we were to receive. In the meantime, the A/C repairman said it would take three days to get the motor shipped to him. Time! Well, we had a good attitude and knew we would have cold air soon.

The point is, being a Victor is for your lifetime, not just for a moment.

Think of it this way, the Chicago Cubs won the World Series in 2016. It had been 108 years since they won a World Series. The city celebrated, the players were heroes, the owners were applauded and exalted. Ten minutes after the champagne was popped, they were asked if they could repeat in 2017. They barely had time to enjoy this one and the expectation for the next year was already thrust upon them. In the summer of 2017, the Cubs were mediocre at best. Their 2016 victory was quickly forgotten. By the end of the summer, they were back on track and they were in contention, but they did not repeat their win in 2017. I am sure that knowing they had been champions and could win helped them rise up and get back on track.

I have been guilty of thinking about a moment of victory and believing that equated to a lifetime of being a Victor. I am not just hitting a goal (like win the World Series or the Super Bowl, lose 100 pounds, etc.) so I can coast or go back to my old ways. I am a Victor for Life and that takes time!

Chapter Review

I suggest you take a few minutes and review the **Ask Yourself** questions and the **Key Points** highlighted in this chapter. Also, take the time to read and meditate on the **scriptures** that helped me on my journey from **Victim** to **Victor**.

Ask Yourself…

Do I see myself maintaining a healthy lifestyle for the rest of my life?

*Am I committed to being a **Victor for Life**?*

Key Points Review:

➢ The key to being committed to being a Victor for Life is to be a Victor one day at a time.

➢ The point is being a Victor is for your lifetime, not just for a moment.

Record what God reveals to you about who He says you are from each of these scriptures. Try reading the verses in different translations of the Bible for even further insight.

1 Corinthians15:52

2 Kings 7:1

PART 5

IM VS. OR

Well, we are heading down the home stretch. We have cruised through the **V**'s, **I**'s, **C**'s, and **T**'s. Let's finish this off discussing the IM of **Victim** vs. the OR of **Victor**. The Bible hero I am focusing on is King David. Certainly, Jesus is the ultimate **Victor**, but most of us are more like King David in the natural than Jesus, so let's see how King David demonstrates a **Victor**'s attitude.

CHAPTER 14

IMMOVABLE MOUNTAIN/ OBTAINABLE REWARDS

VICTIM OR VICTOR, I SEE A CONTRAST IN THE LAST two letters of these words. The "**IM**" causes a Vic**tim** to see challenges as **Immovable Mountains**. The "**OR**" causes a Vic**tor** to see challenges as something to be overcome leading to **Obtainable Rewards**. I know you can see this is really about **attitude**.

When I played football and when I was in basic training in the Army, I heard this phrase often "Get yo' mind right!" **Attitude**. Of course, my whole life's transformation is due to Jesus, who had the ultimate mindset and attitude! The Bible tells us in Philippians 2:5, "Let this mind be in you, which was also in Christ Jesus" (NKJV). Hebrews 12:2 says that Jesus endured the cross, despising the shame for the joy set before Him.

Another classic Bible example is David versus Goliath. In 1 Samuel 17, we read that the whole army of Israel was afraid of Goliath. Saul offered a generous reward to anyone that would defeat/kill Goliath. They all knew what the reward was, but they all viewed Goliath as an **immovable mountain**, rather than seeing the **obtainable reward** for conquering the mountain. On the other hand, David saw it as an opportunity and an **obtainable reward.** He stepped up and killed the giant Goliath, cut his head off, and received the reward.

We can see some important keys to this victory in this story of David versus Goliath in 1 Samuel 17:

1. The most important attitude David had was a complete faith and trust in the power of God to do anything! (See 1 Samuel 17:37.)
2. David's attitude was that God was obligated to fulfill His covenant (Word). (See 1 Samuel 17:45-47.)
3. Another attitude David had was that God would fulfill His covenant with David. (See 1 Samuel 17:34-36.)

I know God can do all things. I am also convinced that God is obligated to fulfill His Word. Now, usually, I believe He will fulfill His Word for Robert Lee Wells Jr. However, there are times I allow doubts about my performance to cause me to doubt if He will do it for me. I know He can do it and I know He will do it, but He might not do it for me because I might not deserve His help or blessing.

Have I prayed enough?
Have I confessed the right scriptures?
Have I confessed them enough times?
Have I sinned? Of course, I have!
Did I confess and receive forgiveness?
Do I deserve to suffer the penalty of my actions? Have I given enough?

Did I obey when God prompted me to tell someone about Jesus?

Ask Yourself…

Does this sound like my attitude?
Do I ask these questions?

David was not worried about his performance. He was so convinced of the goodness, mercy, and love of God that his attitude was that God would do it. I have to remind myself that God really loves me. God actually truly loves me. God so loved **all** Christians that live a perfect life that He gave His only begotten Son, huh, what? Oh, He loved the whole world, all people, even those who don't even know about Him, all the people that know but still want to live in bondage to sin. God loves everybody. He is not happy with sinful behavior, but He is still willing to help me when I ask for help. My attitude is developing into one of knowing His love and trusting His faithfulness.

David knew all this. David recounted some other victories to King Saul that he knew he achieved only because of God's help. So, when this next mountain, Goliath, came up, he had a Victor's attitude. He knew God would help him defeat Goliath and obtain the reward for killing the giant.

I am talking about being a Victor. I am using my weight loss as an example to demonstrate how I made the transition. I recognized that my weight was an outward display of a lazy, selfish, poor-me attitude. I then realized that I could change my attitude. I **could** change **my** attitude with God's help.

Your attitude belongs to **you**! Your attitude will obey **you**! If you blame other people, that's your attitude obeying **you**. If you are afraid of everything, that's your attitude obeying **you**. "Yeah, but they did blah, blah…the terrorist said they were going to blah, blah…people treat me wrong because I'm Black/Mexican/woman/fat/etc." That's your attitude. Oprah Winfrey is a black woman, who openly discusses her struggles with her weight, in a male-dominated industry, and she is one of the wealthiest people in the world. Not just one of the wealthiest women, not just one of the wealthiest black people, one of the wealthiest people…period. Her attitude determined her altitude! You own your attitude!

Chuck Swindoll said, "Your attitude determines your altitude!"[19]

Attitude is a settled way of thinking or feeling about someone or something, typically one that is reflected in a person's behavior; truculent or uncooperative behavior; a resentful or antagonistic manner; individuality and self-confidence as manifested by behavior or appearance; style; the orientation of an aircraft or spacecraft, relative to the direction of travel.[20]

I included the last definition about the orientation of an aircraft because it relates to the quote by Chuck Swindoll. In his illustration about attitude, he explains, "Flight instructors teach that a pilot has to monitor the attitude of the aircraft as carefully as they monitor the altitude of the aircraft."[21] That is where the phrase "your attitude determines your altitude" originated.

The first definition of attitude applies to how I had to deal with my **I**mmovable **M**ountain. I had a settled way of thinking about my weight. For most of my life, I believed I was just supposed to be fat. I was usually chubby, but I was a good athlete, so the only time it mattered was when I liked a girl. Then I would worry that she wouldn't like me because I was fat. I can only remember feeling like I was in good shape when I was a Plebe at West Point and I boxed in my junior year. My attitude was settled that I was fat and I would always be fat. Can you see where this is going? Since I am always going to be fat, why try to lose weight?

I tried to lose weight. I would lose twenty to thirty pounds and then I would feel like I was able to eat what I wanted. My settled way of thinking was I only need to eat this tasteless healthy food for a couple of weeks and then I will be able to get back to the good tasting food. I am sure many of you have a similar settled thought pattern.

Ask Yourself...

Do I have a similar settled thought pattern about my Immovable Mountain?

Here's how the Lord helped me change that settled way of thinking. I was praying and asking God to remove my

Immovable Mountain. I thought if I had a chiseled body like my sons have, I would eat better food. The Lord said, "For Real? Are you serious? Bob, they have chiseled bodies because they eat healthful foods and they workout consistently." It was a paradigm shift. If I ate healthful foods and I increased my work out time, I could have a chiseled body. I saw it!

Instead of eating foods that weakened my heart and at the same time caused my heart to need to work harder, if I ate foods that strengthened my heart and at the same time caused my heart to need to work as designed, I could be healthy. Now, I had to double down with the exercise. If I stopped sitting around which contributed to my heart and muscles getting weaker. Less muscle burns less fat, so you get fatter. Contrast that to just walking thirty minutes per day and my heart got stronger, my leg muscles got stronger, and I was burning fat. Hallelujah!

I hope you can see if you change your settled way of thinking, you can change your life.

Looking at the third definition that attitude is reflected in a person's truculent or uncooperative behavior, I realized I had to change from a style of "Big Bob," "Big Man," "Big Ol' teddy bear," to "Hey Slim," "Man, you gonna disappear," "Dad, I can get my arms all the way around you!" That's the one that got me right there. My kids wanted to hug me, but I didn't know they wanted to put their arms around me. I'm choked up as I type this. Well, praise God, they can still get their arms all the way around me. So, I believe this third definition is what my kids call swag. It's an outward behavior that reflects my inner attitude about myself. Body language often reveals our attitude about ourselves.

When I think about Jesus going into the wilderness to be tempted, He **knew** what He was facing! It wasn't a prompting that the wilderness seemed like a good idea. He knew it was so He could be tested and tried and then tempted. So, Jesus had His mind right and had His "I have the Victory over you Satan" swag!

I had my fat-boy swag. I liked sitting around chillin'. I liked eating extra helpings even when I was full. I liked joking about being fat. I had swag, but it was the wrong kind of swag, the wrong attitude. Now, I have a different swag.

> **It's an, "I know that I am getting healthier" swag.**
> **It's an, "I can do all things through Christ" swag.**
> **It's an, "I'm a 180-pound-man" swag.**

Chapter Review

I suggest you take a few minutes and review the **Ask Yourself** questions and the **Key Points** highlighted in this chapter. Also, take the time to read and meditate on the **scriptures** that helped me on my journey from Victim to Victor.

Ask Yourself...

Is my attitude negatively affecting my altitude?
Do I demonstrate a Victor's attitude?

Ask Yourself...

Does this sound like my attitude? Do I ask these types of questions?

Have I prayed enough?
Have I confessed the right scriptures?
Have I confessed them enough times?
Have I sinned? Of course, I have!
Did I confess and receive forgiveness?
Do I deserve to suffer the penalty of my actions? Have I given enough?
Did I obey when God prompted me to tell someone about Jesus?

Ask Yourself...

Do I have a negative settled thought pattern about my seemingly Immovable Mountain?

What do I have to do to deal with my "settled way of thinking" to become a victor and not a victim?

Ask Yourself...

Do I have the right kind or the wrong kind of swag?
Do I need to change my sway?

Key Points Review:

➤ **Chuck Swindoll said, "Your attitude determines your altitude!"**

➤ **I hope you can see if you change your settled way of thinking, you can change your life.**

Record what God reveals to you about who He says you are from each of these scriptures.

Philippians 2:5
Hebrews 12:2
1 Samuel 17

Final Word

Be Encouraged

I WANT TO ENCOURAGE YOU TO MAKE A QUALITY DECI-sion to advance from **Victim** to **Victor**. This decision will impact every area of your life. I started with my weight and I am moving on to my marriage, my family, my finances, my ministry, etc. I want you to have God's vision for your life.

> ➢ Create your value statement.
> ➢ Guard your mouth and speak life to your vision.
> ➢ Study the Word to find out your true identity in Christ.
> ➢ Get intelligence (wisdom) and make integrity your trademark.
> ➢ Consider the impact of your choices daily and choose life!
> ➢ Demonstrate your commitment by your consistency.
> ➢ Stir up your courage to get started, to keep going, and to finish!
> ➢ Discover or re-discover and appreciate your talents.
> ➢ Expect tests and trials and expect to overcome every test and trial that you face.

➢ Settle it in your heart that being a victor is for a lifetime and be willing to take that much time.

➢ Remember there are no **Immovable Mountains** with God, only His amazing **Obtainable Rewards**

➢ Be a Victor for Life.

I pray you will apply these lessons and join me in living Life as a Victor! God Bless you!

Author Information

Robert "Bob" Wells is a former US Army Officer, a c/o 1987 West Point graduate, husband, and father. Bob has been involved in Men's Ministry since 1994, serving as a Promise Keepers ambassador for the city of Danville, Il for four years. Bob and his wife Cathy have been active in marriage ministry for over twelve years, both in couples' counseling and teaching. Bob currently leads a weekly men's ministry helping men develop a closer walk with the Lord and fulfilling their God-given destinies as Victors in life.

Endnotes

1   https://www.christianquotes.info/quotes-by-topic/
    quotes-about-choices/

2   Merriam-Webster's Collegiate Dictionary, Eleventh
    Edition, © copyright 2009 by Merriam-Webster,
    Incorporated

3   Merriam-Webster's Collegiate Dictionary, Eleventh
    Edition, © copyright 2009 by Merriam-Webster,
    Incorporated

4   Joshua 14:6-14

5   Merriam-Webster's Collegiate Dictionary, Eleventh
    Edition, © copyright 2009 by Merriam-Webster,
    Incorporated

6   Merriam-Webster's Collegiate Dictionary, Eleventh
    Edition, © copyright 2009 by Merriam-Webster,
    Incorporated

7   The Passion Translation (TPT) The Passion
    Translation®. Copyright © 2017 by BroadStreet
    Publishing® Group, LLC. Used by permission. All
    rights reserved. thePassionTranslation.com

[8] Merriam-Webster's Collegiate Dictionary, Eleventh Edition, © copyright 2009 by Merriam-Webster, Incorporated

[9] Merriam-Webster's Collegiate Dictionary, Eleventh Edition, © copyright 2009 by Merriam-Webster, Incorporated

[10] Merriam-Webster's Collegiate Dictionary, Eleventh Edition, © copyright 2009 by Merriam-Webster, Incorporated

[11] Merriam-Webster's Collegiate Dictionary, Eleventh Edition, © copyright 2009 by Merriam-Webster, Incorporated

[12] quotefancy.com/quote/35/Albert-Einstein-Insanity-is-doing-the-same-thing-over-and-over-

[13] quotefancy.com/quote/35/Albert-Einstein-Insanity-is-doing-the-same-thing-over-and-over-

[14] Merriam-Webster's Collegiate Dictionary, Eleventh Edition, © copyright 2009 by Merriam-Webster, Incorporated

[15] Merriam-Webster's Collegiate Dictionary, Eleventh Edition, © copyright 2009 by Merriam-Webster, Incorporated

[16] Merriam-Webster's Collegiate Dictionary, Eleventh Edition, © copyright 2009 by Merriam-Webster, Incorporated

17 Merriam-Webster's Collegiate Dictionary, Eleventh Edition, © copyright 2009 by Merriam-Webster, Incorporated

18 Merriam-Webster's Collegiate Dictionary, Eleventh Edition, © copyright 2009 by Merriam-Webster, Incorporated

19 https://insight.org/resources/daily-devotional/ individual/the-value-of-a-positive-attitude

20 Merriam-Webster's Collegiate Dictionary, Eleventh Edition, © copyright 2009 by Merriam-Webster, Incorporated

21 https://insight.org/resources/daily-devotional/ individual/the-value-of-a-positive-attitude

CPSIA information can be obtained
at www.ICGtesting.com
Printed in the USA
BVHW072129020221
599232BV00010B/213

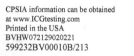